C000225919

Black Seed Oil

The Effect of Black Seed Oil Against Cancer

(The Therapeutic Effect of Black Seed Oil on Rheumatoid Arthritis)

Lydia Tennant

Published By **Jackson Denver**

Lydia Tennant

Black Seed Oil: The Effect of Black Seed Oil Against Cancer (The Therapeutic Effect of Black Seed Oil on Rheumatoid Arthritis)

ISBN 978-1-77485-759-5

No part of this guidebook shall be reproduced in any form without permission in writing from the publisher except in the case of brief quotations embodied in critical articles or reviews.

Legal & Disclaimer

The information contained in this ebook is not designed to replace or take the place of any form of medicine or professional medical advice. The information in this ebook has been provided for educational & entertainment purposes only.

The information contained in this book has been compiled from sources deemed reliable, and it is accurate to the best of the Author's knowledge; however, the Author cannot guarantee its accuracy and validity and cannot be held liable for any errors or omissions. Changes are periodically made to this book. You must consult your doctor or get professional medical advice before using any of the suggested remedies, techniques, or information in this book.

Upon using the information contained in this book, you agree to hold harmless the Author from and against any damages, costs, and expenses, including any legal fees potentially resulting from the application of any of the information provided by this guide. This disclaimer applies to any damages or injury caused by the use and application, whether directly or indirectly, of any advice or information presented, whether for breach of contract, tort, negligence, personal injury, criminal intent, or under any other cause of action.

You agree to accept all risks of using the information presented inside this book. You need to consult a professional medical practitioner in order to ensure you are both able and healthy enough to participate in this program.

TABLE OF CONTENTS

Introduction

There are plenty of natural remedies that have an extensive history of use that have been neglected in the last few years. From hair- and health increasing components of castor oils to the alternative remedy made using Apple Cider Vinegar, treatments that are found in nature perform important functions for keeping your health in good shape.

Many doctors, including medicinal and naturopathic doctors, are successful when they combine orthodox medical practices with natural techniques to help the body. One of these treatments that is gaining recent acceptance is Black Seed Oil or Nigella Sativa.

Due to the amazing advancements in medicine and hygiene many of these treatments are neglected. There's certain to be a time and a place in medical research, however it has helped to understand the processes behind the natural remedies that people from the past have relied on for a long time.

The black, small and thick-shaped seed is often referred to as "black seeds" or "black cumin seeds'. They're a little curly with rough texture on their outside , which makes them distinct and easy to identify. They originate from The Nigella Sativa Flower and can be grown in all parts of the world.

Oil is extracted from black seeds by pressing and pressing the seeds. There are many big home appliances that can aid in the creation of the oil, or purchase it as oil. The oil is a powerful and intense flavor.

The drug and its many possibilities of use have an element of host that makes it efficient in the body to treat various ailments and illnesses. For more than 2000 years this plant has been utilized in medical treatments and was found within the burial site of Tutankhamun in Egypt. From the time of ancient times the black seed was utilized to treat toothaches, headaches and nasal congestion. It's also known to treat conjunctivitis (the pink eye) as well as parasites and abscesses (pockets of infection).

Digestive tract disorders like dysentery, diarrhoea hemorrhoids, constipation and diarrhoea are treated with black seeds today. As well, medical conditions such as asthma and allergies, swine influenza and emphysema. Congestion and bronchitis congestion are treated by the black seed. Women are also reported using the black seeds to control birth to increase the flow of milk and to begin menstrual flow.

There's a lot the black seed has to offer not just internally, but externally too. The next chapters will help open your eyes to a world of possibilities regarding the benefits on Black Seed Oil in your appearance and health! This will provide you with an entire range of information on Black Seed Oil. We thank you for embarking on this journey along with me.

Chapter 1: What Is Black Seed And Black Seed Oil?

Black Cumin Seed Oil Black Cumin Seed Oil which is sometimes referred to Black Coriander Oil or simply Black Oil comes from the Nigella Sativa plant which is native to Asia. Recent studies on this powerful seed oil suggest it can be useful in fighting superbugs such as MRSA or h.pylori and cancer patients.

The plant is part of the buttercup family . It is a small black crescent-shaped seeds. Black seed reports in the past of its usage date back as early as the reign that of King Tut and his cronies in Ancient Egypt. It is said that Cleopatra was said to have used the oil of black cumin seeds for gorgeous skin and hair, and Hippocrates loved using it to treat issues related to stomach.

Archaeologists have even discovered black seeds inside King Tut's tomb. This highlights their importance in the past to protection and healing. They are also used to flavor curries, breads as well as pickles. When consumed they always have an unpleasant taste that is frequently compared to oregano or cumin.

A few other names for black seed oil are the following: black caraway cumin and black onion seeds. Kalonji.

There are over 600 studies that have proven the benefits of the black cumin seed oil. There are ongoing studies on the benefits in black cumin seeds oil in treating autoimmune diseases. The active components crystallized nigellone and thymoquinone are the most extensively studied and studied, however it also contains palmitic acid, palmitoleic acid myristic acidand stearic acid Oleic acid, Linoleic acid arachidonic acids, protein and vitamins B1 and B2 as well as B3 folate, calcium, iron copper, zinc, and phosphorus.

The oil of black seed is made by removing the seeds from the black cumin (Nigella sativa) plant which is part of the ranunculus family (Ranunculaceae). Black cumin is indigenous to the southwest of Asia as well as in the Mediterranean as well as Africa. It is grown for a long time because of its aromatic, scent and tasty seeds. It is utilized in the form of spices or as an herbal remedy. Black seed oil is frequently referred to as black cumin oil. It is essential to be cautious, as black seed shouldn't be confused with genuine cumin (Cuminum Cyminum) and black pepper. black cohosh or black sesame.

Perhaps the most exciting research has been conducted connecting Nigella sativa to multi-drug-resistant bacteria. This is a huge deal as these "superbugs" are now becoming a major health risk for the general public.

The study, which was carried out by Jawaharlal Nehru Medical College researchers set out to find out how effective black seed oil is against superbugs. They also compared it with various antibiotics, including Amoxicillin, Gatifloxacin and Tetracycline. The study found that "Out from 144 bacteria that were tested, the majority of them were resistant to a variety of antibiotics, just 97 were inhibited due to the oil from black cumin."

The most important reason to understand why black seed oils benefit the body in this manner is that it's high in three important natural chemical compounds such as Thymoquinone (TQ) and the thymohydroquinone (THQ) and Thymol. Let's look closer at the amazing ingredients of the black seed oil.

The Power of Black Seed oil benefits: Phytochemicals

In an effort to provide an answer to the increasing resistance to antifungal that people experience with molds and yeasts the researchers conducted a study to determine whether Nigella sativa seeds oil might aid. The study was published within the Egyptian Journal of Biochemistry & Molecular Biology researchers examined thymol, TQ, and THQ against 30 pathogens in humans and were shocked to discover that

* Each compound demonstrated 100 percent inhibition against the 30 pathogens that were tested

Thymoquinone was found to be the most effective antifungal ingredient against all the yeasts and dermatophytes tested that were tested, followed by thymohydroquinone as well as Thymol.

THYMOOL was the most effective antifungal for molds, which was followed by TQ and then THQ.

What this study shows us is that Nigella Sativa oil has the unique chemical component that is not just effective as a whole, but it is also effective for a whole collection of individuals. In essence, it proves that fungus and molds can't exist with these phytochemicals, there is the reason why scientists are looking to find a solution to the superbug issue using the black seed oil.

Thymoquinone Researchers say that who have been studying TQ from the 60s. It is an active ingredient found in the black seed. It is well-known due to it's antioxidant, anti-inflammatory, and anticancer properties . It has been reported to help with the encephalomyelitis, carcinogenesis and diabetes as well as asthma.

Interestingly, thymoquinone acts as a free radical or an effective superoxide radical scavenger, in addition to preserving antioxidant enzymes glutathione peroxidase and glutathione-S-transferase. Both S-transferase and glutathione peroxidase are widely regarded as significant detoxifiers, and are a major part of antioxidant defense mechanisms in cells as they shield the liver from the effects of toxins.

Thymohydroquinone is similar to thymoquinone of the most powerful naturally occurring the acetylcholinesterase (AChE) inhibitors found on the globe. The AChE inhibitors are chemical compounds which block enzyme activity. increasing the amount of time of the neurotransmitter, acetylcholine, that is active within the brain. The pharmaceutical-grade acetylcholinesterase inhibitors can be utilized to treat a variety of illnesses. The following is an example of their effectiveness:

The disease of Apathy Dementia or Alzheimer's diseases. Neurodegenerative disorders, Autism, Postural tachycardia syndrome, Glaucoma Parkinson's disease Schizophrenia.

When considering the approach of pharmaceuticals to these illnesses, it could result in a significant cost for patients. Black seed oil, however, offers an abundance of hope to many because it's an effective, safe and plant-based solution and alternative to numerous.

Thymol: This is the primary ingredient that enables thyme essential oil to be used in its therapeutic qualities. Thymol is a monoterpene natural that has a range of beneficial properties. For instance:

* It is typically employed as a virucides or tuberculocidal in order to kill TB and other virus.

* It's an general-purpose and medical disinfectant.

This is quick degradingand non-persistent insecticide.

* Used to flavor food items or perfumes, mouthwashes, fragrances and even cosmetics

* These amazing phytochemicals contribute to a myriad of fantastic benefits from black seed oil

It may not look exactly like the way you've seen it or are familiar with, but these trees produce fruits with small black seeds. The seeds of black were used to treat ailments throughout the ages.

Chapter 2: Benefits Of The Oil From The Black Seed

Black oil seeds have been proven to treat a variety of most prevalent health issues as well as rare ailments such as hypertension and asthma. It's also been found to show a high degree of antifungal properties against Candida albicans, yeast, which causes candidiasis when it grows within the body.

Of the many ways that the black seed oil can benefit the body There are a few that stand out in the world of science for example, such as its capability to reduce the risk of weight gain as well as hair loss, cancer skin diseases, diabetes and infections such as MRSA.

There are numerous health benefits associated with the oil from the black seeds in greater detail, including:

1. Fighting Cancer

The oil from the black seed is believed to aid in combat cancer due to the potent phytochemicals it contains and its antioxidant properties and capabilities. The study looked at the antitumor effects of thymoquinone as well as

Thymohydroquinone has been discovered was discovered by Croatian researchers by using an animal model. Ut was also found that the two phytochemicals, which are present in the black seed oil caused the reduction by 52 percent within tumor cells.

Recent studies over the years have revealed that hydroquinone is one of the bioactive ingredient in the oil from the black seeds aids in triggering the process of apoptosis (programmed the death of cells) on breast cancer cells and brain tumor cells, as in Leukemia cells. Researchers at The Sidney Kimmel Cancer Center at Jefferson Health have revealed that black seeds can kill pancreatic cancer cells , and is believed to hinder the growth of pancreatic cancer. This ability to prevent cancer is an outcome of black seed's Thymoquinone as well as its anti-inflammatory properties.

2. Helps Improve Liver Health

The liver is among the most vital organs in the human body. The majority of toxins are removed from the body due to the the liver.

The bile that is produced by the liver is crucial to digesting fats and aiding your body to stay healthy and happy.

If you've been suffering from a weak liver as a result of negative effects from medications or diseases, or an excessive consumption of alcohol you will discover that black seed oil to increase the speed of healing. In a recent animal study, researchers discovered that black seed oil aids in the prevention of the development of diseases and damage to the liver.

3. Combats Diabetes

Researchers from the Indian Council of Medical Research assert that the oil of black seeds induces gradual partial development of pancreatic beta-cells. It raises insulin levels, and also reduces increased levels of glucose in the bloodstream. This is the result of an article recently published by the Journal of Endocrinology and Metabolism. This is amazing because Nigella Sativa is one of the very few ingredients in the world that aids in the prevention of type 1 diabetes and type.

In this report the black seed can improve tolerance to glucose as effectively as metformin. Despite this, it hasn't shown any significant negative effects and is low toxic effects. This is important due to the fact that metformin is one of the most frequently prescribed drugs for type 2 diabetes is associated with a broad spectrum of adverse reactions, which include:

Gas/indigestion

Skin blemishes

Heartburn

Bloating

Nail changes

Constipation/diarrhoea

Headache

Stomach pain

4. Helps with Weight Loss

A study was published in The Journal of Diabetes and Metabolic Disorders. The study suggests that the black seed oil's weight loss does actually have certain scientific proof behind them as they systematically reviewed the research to find the plants that possess anti-obesity properties. The researchers found it was true that the oil of black seeds is among some of the best natural cures available on the world.

The study was published in 2018 and is yet another meta-analysis, systematic study and systematic reviews that focuses on the findings of at the very least 11 placebo-controlled clinical studies and mistakes, that revealed the capacity of the supplement with black seeds to aid in reducing body weight. It was also found that the Body Mass Index (BMI) and waist circumference was as well reduced with supplementation. It is important to note that there were not adverse side effects associated with supplementation with black seed in any study.

6. Provides treatment for Infections (MRSA)

Methicillin-resistant staphylococcus aureus, commonly referred to in the form (MRSA) is among the most significant Superbugs black seed oil is able to eliminate. MRSA is found in every hospital and nursing homes across the world because Staph infections are getting resistant to antibiotics that are used internally.

The older age group is more susceptible to the disease due to the fact that it is usually connected to procedures such as surgery, intravenous tubing or artificial joints. Senior citizens has created MRSA an international public health risk, primarily because of their weaker immunity.

It's great to know that the health benefits of black oils can aid in reducing the risk of this disease. Researchers from Pakistan tested several varieties of MRSA and discovered that each was sensitive to black seeds which indicates that the oil could help to reduce and even stop MRSA from spreading.

7. Improves Fertility

To add to the potential of aiding in the fight against the superbugs that plague us, there's many other things that black seed oil could aid in, such as its capacity to boost fertility naturally. A controlled, placebo-controlled double-blind, controlled clinical trial examined whether or not black seed oil can help males who are infertile by using fake male sperm. The participants took in .5 milliliters (milliliters) of oil from black seeds orally. The placebo group took the equivalent amount of liquid paraffin over a period of two months two times a day. What was found? It was discovered that the people who were in the group of black seed oil were able to increase their sperm count and the volume of sperm and the motility of sperm.

8. Balances Cholesterol and Balances

Yes! The oil from the black seed also provides benefits in relation to managing cholesterol levels. Based on an animal model an article published in 2007 revealed that an aqueous extract of Nigella Sativa had anti-diabetic effects on animals and also helped fight cholesterol levels. Following six weeks of providing small doses of black seed oil to diabetic animals the glucose, total cholesterol levels were all reduced. LDL cholesterol, and HDL cholesterol was elevated.

The consumption of oil from seeds is believed to lower high cholesterol. It's rich in healthy fatty acids that assist in maintaining a healthy cholesterol level. Examples of these acids are the linoleic acid and oleic acid. The place in which the seeds are planted can affect the amount of oil. The results will be evident when eating the seeds crushed.

9. Asthma and Allergies

The oils of black seed are believed to possess anti-asthmatic benefits and, dependent on the underlying cause of asthma it can be more effective than traditional treatment, as per reports from many studies. These same ingredients can be beneficial in helping to reduce allergies in many people.

Asthma symptoms can be greatly improved by the anti-inflammatory benefits of the black seed oil. It can also aid in reducing asthma symptoms.

10. Heart Health

It is believed that the presence Thymoquinone found in Nigella Sativa seeds is proven to provide a protection for the heart. This helps to maintain good cholesterol levels, and reduce blood pressure.

11. Immune Health

It is Nigella Sativa is unique in its approach to aiding our immune system. It is a rich source of antioxidants, beneficial acids and b-vitamins which aid in strengthening the immune system, but it does so differently from herbs like echinacea or the elderberry , which should be avoided by those suffering from an autoimmune condition. There is a significant amount of equilibrium of the immune system - the improvement of immune function through black seeds has been reported but it is not encouraging immune reactions against healthy tissue in the body.

It has also been utilized in other HIV treatment protocols for many years. It is frequently advised on forums dealing with autoimmune diseases (with testimonials from people that it has helped).

12. Digestion

It is believed that Nigella Sativa seeds are carminative. They aid with digestion and could reduce gas stomach pain, bloating and stomach pain. The oil from the black seed is often used as a remedy to treat intestinal parasites. When studied, it has been proven to slow tumor growth in colon cancer and has no adverse side effects.

13. Candida and Fungus

The oil of black seed is well-known for its effectiveness in fighting and eliminating fungal and candida-related illnesses in the digestive tract and also for the appearance of the skin. It helps to restore balance to your body, and also eliminate candida.

Other benefits of oil from the black seed are:

* Lowering blood pressure: The continuous consumption of extracts from black cumin seeds for a period of two months and beyond has been shown to lower high blood pressure in those who have blood pressure that is moderately elevated or slightly elevated.

Improved symptoms of rheumatoid arthritis by taking a single dose of black seed oil can assist in reducing inflammation symptoms of rheumatoid.

* Reducing stomach upsets The oil from black seeds as well as eating black seeds can be associated with easing stomach pain and cramps. The oil aids in reducing gas and the possibility of stomach ulcers, as well as gastric bloating, and.

Black seed oil in the form of potions called thymoquinone as well as other potions of seeds could be used to slow down the development of tumors in laboratory rats. The oil can also assist in reducing the harmful consequences of radiation utilized to kill cancerous cells. However, these findings haven't yet been tested on our bodies. The oil from black seeds shouldn't be used to substitute for traditional cancer treatments.

Overall, it's evident that the black seed and its oil can aid in lowering cholesterol levels as also blood sugar levels and blood pressure. The benefits of this seed are endless.

Chapter 3: The Aspects That Can Be Averted By Black Seed Oil

Black seed oil has numerous benefits that it's hard to imagine any negative side effects. But, we all know that each oil has its own setbacks. There are issues with any seed, vegetable or oil, which includes the oil from black cumin seeds when it's not processed, extracted or packaged correctly. It is likely to spoil when any of these steps are not adhered to. It is essential that the oil is kept in a dark transparent glass container (preferably the miron type).

What to look for in the Black Cumin Seed Oil:

It is the Black Cumin Seed Oil is the best absorbable, concentrated and absorbent form that is also the most efficient method to consume black seeds. It's just essential to ensure it comes from a reliable source, and most importantly organic, and purely extracted without chemical extraction, and without additives or diluting oils, secured from rancidity with high quality light and air-protection glass.

The oil extracted from black cumin seeds could be food item that contains certain concentrated substances that might not be as effective. As with all food items be sure to ensure that whatever type of product you choose is of high-quality and free of harmful additives.

Breastfeeding and pregnancy:

A substantial amount of black seeds appears to be safe to eat in small quantities during pregnancy. If you are taking a higher quantity, it's likely to be dangerous since it may slow down or prevent the uterus from expanding during labor. There isn't much information about how to utilize the black seed while nursing, so it's advised to be in the safe zone and avoid using. According to Memorial Sloan-Kettering Cancer Center, pregnant women shouldn't consume black seeds in any way. A further examination is required to know exactly how this may affect pregnancy, therefore it is recommended to stay clear of the substance if you are expecting a baby.

Children Black seeds are possible to be safe for children when it is taken orally in short-term and in the recommended doses of small amounts.

Bleeding disorders: The dark seed could actually slow down bleeding, and may increase the chance of bleeding. Also, the black seeds can make bleeding disorder worse. Make sure to consult your physician prior to using when you have an issue with bleeding.

Diabetes: Be aware of indications for low levels of blood sugar (hypoglycemia) since the black seed can reduce blood sugar levels in certain individuals. Be aware of your blood sugar levels in case you suffer from diabetes and are considering using the oil.

Hypotension A: The Memorial Sloan-Kettering Cancer Center advices to avoid this, especially if you're taking diuretics or antihypertensive medication and the black seed could reduce blood pressure until the level of hypotension. The decrease in blood pressure prevents the delivery for oxygen and nutrients to your brain, the heart and other organs. It can result in weak breathing, fatigue blurred vision, dizziness, nausea, lightheadedness as well as loss of conscious. If blood pressure drops too low, it could be life-threatening.

Tiredness and Drowsiness People recommend the oil of black seeds to aid in sleeping. Some people have found that using the oil of black seed, it made them feel exhausted during work hours or they felt sleepy. Certain people felt more tired than they normally are. If this is the case for you take a break from how much black seeds you're taking, or quit completely to prevent any kind of accident.

Surgery Black seeds are well-known to decrease blood clotting, decrease blood sugar levels, and cause sleepiness in some individuals. This is why it is crucial to be aware that the use of the black seed can increase the risk of bleeding, affect blood sugar control , and cause anesthesia following any surgery. It is recommended to avoid the use of the black seeds within two weeks in advance of the scheduled procedure.

Contact dermatitis: Another result from the seed's black color is contact skin rashes. Simply touching the black seeds, you can trigger a severe red rash that covers the skin of certain people and is often followed by a sensation of itching. The rash can also lead to the appearance of blisters, pain, or tenderness just to the site that is exposed.

Negative Interactions:

Based on research conducted by the Memorial Sloan-Kettering Cancer Center, the black seed is associated with adverse interactions with chemotherapy drugs and radiation. This herb can reduce the effectiveness of standard treatment for cancer since it can be an antioxidant within the body.

Other Allergic Reactions

In comparison to nearly every herbal remedy, there's the possibility of an allergic reaction resulting from consumption. In contrast to the contact dermatitis side result, this allergic reaction doesn't just affect the skin. It could create swelling in the face, tongue and throat, lips or and difficulty breathing or breathing, a sensation of tingling in the tongue, nausea nausea as well as vomiting, diarrhea and abdominal pains that are a result of the stomach.

For certain people, black cumin can cause an allergic reaction when inhaled and applied on the face. Before applying black cumin essential oil applied topically it is recommended to conduct a patch test to ensure you do not have a allergic reaction. Avoid eye contact and mucous membranes whenever applying black seed oil.

If swallowed by mouth, the oil of black seeds causes stomach bloating and vomiting or constipation. Certain individuals could cause seizure risk.

Like any essential oil, be sure that you keep the black seed oil from light and heat, and out of access of children.

The black seed oil can be very beneficial when it comes down to the liver's function, but using greater amounts of black seed oil that is recommended could cause harm to your kidneys and liver. If you are experiencing any problems regarding either organ discuss it with your physician to determine the appropriate dosage. Additionally, the topical application of black seed oil could trigger allergic reaction. Be sure to conduct an initial patch test prior to applying it to a large part on your face.

It is highly likely that the oil extracted from black seeds can boost the effect of drugs that the body processes via the Cytochrome P450 pathway. The enzymes in this pathway can are able to metabolize 90% of all fundamental medicines. Examples of these medications include beta-blockers, such as metoprolol (Lopressor) as well as blood thinner, warfarin (Coumadin).

If you use any of these medication regularly, consult your physician prior to starting to consume black seed oil for food. Do not take any medication you are taking regularly without speaking to your doctor first.

Chapter 4: Applying The Black Seed Oil To Improve Your Health And Beauty.

In a study in the field of research conducted by experts from Iran in Iran, Nigella Sativa was discovered to be as effective the cream for skin Betamethasone in improving the quality of life and reducing the severity of hand eczema. So long as you do not suffer from allergies to oil of the black seed the oil is not accompanied with a long list of frightening side effects, like other creams.

For instance, Betamethasone, may actually cause a swelling on your hands or face as well as tingling or swelling of your throat or mouth as well as chest tightness, difficulty breathing, changes in the color of your skin dark freckles, bruises, muscle weakness and extreme concentration. The increase in weight around your neck or upper back, and around your waist or breasts. It is among the locations that is thought to be possible.

Hair Benefits

As well as acting as an effective natural skin care aid in addition, there are numerous benefits of black seed oil for the hair. It is not surprising that the oil from black seeds

31

is often listed on lists of ways to improve the condition of hair and scalp in many ways. Since it's a rich source of nigellone which has been proven to be a potent boost to hair health, it could aid in reducing hair loss caused by androgenic alopecia, or Alopecia areata. Due to its antioxidant, antibacterial as well as anti-inflammatory qualities, it could aid in reducing dandruff and dryness, as well as improve the health of your hair at the same time, improving the condition of your scalp overall. This will encourage growth of hair.

The oil from the black seed offers a variety of benefits and applications for the most difficult skin problems. It is available in many health food shops and pharmacy stores. Some examples of how to apply the oil from the black seed on your skin and beauty are:

Acne: According the journal of Dermatology and Dermatologic Surgery, once applying a cream to your body, which is formulated with the black seeds of 10 percent, this significantly reduces the appearance of acne within two months. Participants in the study reported a satisfaction rate of 67 percent.

Hair hydration Black seed oil can be applied to human hair so that it gets soft and improves shine.

Psoriasis: By applying oils made of black, it's been reported to lower the chance of developing plaques of psoriasis.

Skin softening Black seed oil is added to moisturizers and oils to increase the hydration and moisture of skin.

Oil pulling is the use of black seed oil. It was used for oil pulling. The practice of oil pulling can be described as a technique to remove toxins from your body.

Treatment of wounds use Black seed oil is recognized to decrease inflammation and also the amount of bacteria that aid in healing wounds. This single act can stimulate other growth factors and assist the body to create new healthy, beautiful skin.

Remember, never forget that the oil from black seeds isn't a substitute for the official prescription treatments your doctor might provide you with. However, it has some advantages for beauty that complement the treatments that can improve your skin!

Chapter 5: Hypertension

Arterial hypertension is one of the most common diseases among our population. The condition is often not cause any harm and has no symptoms, yet it gradually harms the cardiovascular system and heart. It is a major risk factor for heart disease such as myocardial infarction, heart failure and myocardial infarction as well as strokes or chronic renal failure.

Because hypertension is a lifestyle connected disease, adjustments to diet are crucial in its prevention and management. Oil extracted from black seeds is diet supplement that can lower blood pressure for hypertensive patients even in patients who do not have prescription drug therapy.

The anti-hypertensive effect that black seeds oil exhibits can be seen in the main component of the oil thymoquinone. Its antioxidant action blocks mediator-induced hypertension within blood vessels, and is also a cardio depressant within the nervous system's central part. Additionally, thymoquinone decreases heart rate, thereby providing an additional cardio-protection function.

Other mechanisms also play a role in the regulation of blood pressure. Fats that have unsaturated fats, particularly Oleic, and Linoleic alter the vascular endothelium on the cellular level. This leads to relaxation of the arterial wall and blood pressure decrease. Black seed oil has the effects of a moderate diuretic which is similar to the diuretic drugs that we are used to. It enhances urinary excretion of sodium as well as potassium and water, and relieves the body of fluid by doing this.

Studies have shown that the dosage required to achieve anti-hypertensive effects is between 100 and 200 mg, which is equivalent to one teaspoon of black seeds oil, twice daily for a duration that is at least 8 consecutive weeks.

Diabetes

Achieving a proper control of blood sugar levels of diabetics is essential for lessening the risk of artery damage within the body and the potential developing other complications of diabetes. The conventional anti-diabetic treatment is not achieving the same results in controlling blood sugar levels and metabolic irregularities developing. Because of this, natural solutions that work as a nutritional supplement and help control diabetes are now more popular than ever before.

Patients with diabetes can benefit from the use of black seed oil for diabetics. While it isn't able replace insulin injections, but it has a positive impact on the regulation of glucose levels in type 1 and type 2 diabetics. Black seed oil can stimulate pancreatic cells to make and release more insulin from the endogenous. The tissues in the peripheral region are also more likely to become more sensitive insulin. The glucose is absorbed from blood to cells. Oil extracted from black seeds has been proven that it can affect sugar absorption in the mucosa of the intestine, and it also inhibits gluconeogenesis within the liver. This is a method of making sugar from various organic compounds.

Control of blood sugar levels over time for diabetics is measured by the amount of hemoglobin glycated, also known as hemoglobin A1c or the shorter HbA1c. This indicator shows significant lower levels among diabetics who regularly make use of black seeds oil.

There is evidence to suggest that the anti-diabetic qualities of the oil of black seeds can be attained by drinking 1/2 to 1 teaspoon oil every day for of no less than three months.

Asthma and allergies

The primary pathophysiologic reason for allergic reactions is centered in the home molecule called histamine. The molecule is released by special immune cells known as mast cells when they encounter foreign pathogens. After release, histamine starts the chain reaction, resulting in an overexaggerated and uneffective immune response that causes damage more than it does good.

Black seed oil has the ability to block the release of histamine by mast cells, and stop the chain reaction in the very beginning, thus securing the body from this molecular inflammation. This is because of the metabolite thymoquinone as well as nigell. Why is nigellone important? Remember you've heard the Latin word of Black seed? It's Nigella sativa.

The oil of black seed is extremely powerful against allergies to inhalation like Hay fever, which is the most prevalent kind of allergic disorder. It is caused by allergens, such as pollen or animal feces that are carried through the air by the wind. These particles are taken in by inhalation and then come into contact with the respiratory mucosa and immune system. Thymoquinone as well as nigellone exert powerful effects on mast cells within the respiratory mucosa. These substances reduce the release of histamine. This is why black seed oil has a effective effect against allergic rhinitis. It eases symptoms such as itching, sneezing or a runny nose and congestion in the nose. It does this without adverse effects in local antibody. Studies have shown that black seed oil reduces symptoms in people suffering from allergic rhinitis.

Bronchial asthma can be described as a distinct disease that affects the "lower" regions in the respiratory tract. It is a genetic disease that is caused by the inhalation of allergens and through exposure to other triggers such as tobacco smoke, infection as well as environmental pollutants. The most significant pathological characteristic of asthmatics are inflammations of airways in the small lungs The majority of the medications used in treatment of the disease aim to decrease the severity of this condition. Thus, the reason for prophylactic effects of the oil black seed on asthma is the suppression influence on the inflammation of the small airways. The oil causes dilatation in the bronchial passage and enhances the removal of mucus, thereby improving the function of the lungs. This is the same process that is used by medications like salbutamol or theophylline, both of which are used in the traditional asthma treatment.

Black seed oil has the ability to lessen the frequency of asthma attacks for asthmatics and also relieve symptoms such as wheezing, coughing and breath shortness. Additionally, its use has been shown to improve lung function test results not just in asthmatics but also in those with chronic obstructive bronchitis as well as emphys.

To treat asthma and allergies For the treatment of asthma and allergies, black seed oil can be taken via mouth. It is recommended in an amount of 1 teaspoon twice daily. It should be taken for at least 2 months to show a clear therapeutic benefit. The only exception to this regular use is skin allergies and eczema for which topical application of the face is suggested.

Infections

Black seed oil exhibits the ability to fight off bacteria. It is used to fight illnesses since the ancient times. Modern technological advancements of the technology have enabled us to examine and verify the antibacterial properties from the oil not just in a laboratory ("in in vitro") as well as in the human body ("in in vivo"). The inhibition of bacterial growth and reproduction can be attributed to two key active components of the black seed oils: thymoquinone as well as melanin.

The oil has an impact on two major types of bacteria that are Gram positive as well as Gram negative but having a slight effect for Gram negative. The most vulnerable bacteria to the black seed oil are Staphylococcus aureus, the most frequent cause of throat and skin infections as well as Escherichia coli, which is a well-known source of extremely difficult and painful UTIs. The strength of the antibacterial effects of the black seed oil is comparable to that of antibiotics however in certain instances it is more so. Certain studies have demonstrated the bactericidal effects that black seeds oil has microorganisms resistant more commonly used antibiotics.

In addition to the presence of bacteria Black seed oil is very effective against Candida albicans as well as various fungal diseases. It is a great option for candidiasis treatment for a variety of organs, including throat and mouth infections to parenchymatous organs such as the liver, spleen and kidneys.

The virus is also affected by the black seed oil. It helps alleviate symptoms and decreases the "viral load" in people suffering from viral infection caused by hepatitis viruses and Cytomegalovirus.

To have the greatest antimicrobial effects it is recommended to take one tablespoon of black seeds oil per day. It is ideal to consume early in the morning, before breakfast. It is important to note the fact that oil from black seeds doesn't require the simultaneous taking antibiotics to fight infection, therefore the potential for toxicity from antibiotics is prevented. This is an important aspect to consider when it comes to antimicrobial resistance suppression in the all populations.

Digestive problems

Black seed oil has long been utilized to aid in digestion. Insomnia and loss of appetite can be solved with the help of many of the oil's beneficial components. In acute digestive issues, such as nausea vomiting, nausea and, in particular, diarrhea can be successfully treated using the oil of black seeds.

One of the benefits of the oil black seed is especially important in its healing properties for ulcers caused by peptic. The use of black seed oil can help repair the balance between the protective and aggressive factors within the stomach, the primary mechanism behind the development of ulcers. The oil has been proven effective in Helicobacter pylori elimination, which is the bacteria that causes the development of peptic ulcers. The oil also has properties that protect for the mucosa of the gastric tract that are similar as proton pump inhibitors the medicines commonly employed to protect stomachs. It protects against injuries to mucosa caused through microbial, mechanical, or chemical elements like strong alkalis or ethanol.

The best remedy for digestion problems is to consume one tablespoon of oil from black seeds in the morning, and one in the evening immediately bringing relief and complete recovery in just several days.

Hepatitis

Liver isn't referred to as "body's laboratory" due to accident. It is a repository for all kinds of harmful substances and toxic molecules, then converts them to non-active compounds and eliminates them of the harmful substances. For this reason, the liver is one of the most durable organs in the body. It's not really brittle areas, but Hepatitis virus, which cannot be able to survive for even a moment outside of the body's environment, has the potential of causing irreparable damage to the liver. After being infected with the virus it transforms the liver into the state of chronic illness which is highly resistant to treatment with medications and more prone to further degradation which can lead to liver cirrhosis as well as cancer.

It is extremely efficient in protecting the liver from the hepatitis virus, which is primarily Hepatitis C and Hepatitis B subtypes, which are the most deadly. The primary cause of hepatitis virus-related toxicity is the oxidative stress. This is where antioxidants from black seed oil are put to application. Anti-inflammatory and antioxidant effects that the oil has are the principal properties that protect the liver from damage. You've guessed it: Thymoquinone is the main active ingredient that is responsible for this!

Patients suffering from Hepatitis C infection may take black seed oil along with the usual prescribed medications. It functions as an hepatoprotective. This means that it shields liver cells from pathogens. Consuming oil helps fight the infection and delay the progression of Hepatitis C complications related to the virus such as liver cirrhosis, and cancer. Research has shown that oil consumption decreases "viral burden" and enhances the liver's function. Biochemical parameters of blood aspartate transaminase, alanine transaminas and lactate dehydrogenase have shown an improvement in these parameters when using the oil of black seeds.

For maximum benefit in the hepatitis patient, which is an important improvement in the clinical condition Black seed oil has to be utilized for 3 months at a time and positive results being observed after two weeks of usage.

Tumors

Due to the antioxidant properties of black seed oil it has the ability to eliminate harmful free radicals which could be able to cause pathological alteration of normal cell to an aggressive clone that grows rapidly. Because of this, black seed oil is recommended as a treatment to reduce the risk of tumors.

Black seed oil blocks the growth of tumor cells and is even capable of killing specific kinds of cancer cells. There are various ways of action that contribute to the anti-cancer benefits of the black seed oil. It disrupts the cancer cells' life cycle and stops their growth. It is also adept at activating tumor cells Apoptosis. This is an expression used to describe programmed and induced cell death. Furthermore, anti-cancer activities are evident through the alteration of multiple molecule on cancer cell membranes which makes these cells more susceptible for an immune response. Thymoquinone hinders the growth of blood vessels within the tumor (angiogenesis) and thus limiting the growth of tumors. Metastasis of malignant tumors is slow in certain kinds of tumors.

Black seed oil is producing positive results in many types of cancer. Breast cancer, lung cancer as well as cervical cancer are among the most prevalent human pathology tumors that are impacted by the black seed oil. The oil is anti-cancer and works on tumors of the digestive system, such as liver carcinoma, pancreatic carcinoma and colorectal cancer. It's also effective against skin tumors such as Squamous Cell Carcinoma and malignant melanomas. Recent studies suggest that a benefits of black seed oil could be attained in blood malignancies, specifically lymphomas and leukemia.

Patients who undergo treatment with radiation as a method of treatment for cancer are advised to utilize black seed oilsince it has radioprotective effects on tissues around them that can also be affected by the an oxidative stress caused by ionizing x-ray radiation.

Oil extracted from black seeds is suggested as an adjuvant treatment for patients suffering from tumors. It should be used in conjunction with traditional chemotherapy, and particularly radiotherapy to maximize the effects over time. It is best to consume it regularly 1 teaspoon twice a day.

Neurological disorders

Black seed oil has been proven to be a powerful stimulant for the Central nervous system activities. The mechanism behind the neuropharmacological function of the black seed oil occurs via the modulation of GABA (Gamma-AminoButyric Acid) receptors in the brain. GABA is considered to be the principal inhibitory neurotransmitter within the human brain, whose primary purpose is to decrease excitability of the neuronal system. Black seed oil improves GABA signaling, and it is even believed to boost GABA concentration by itself.

In addition, it enhances the action by increasing the effect of GABA within the brain Black seed oil increases the effect of GABA in the brain. It is able to reduce seizures in epilepsy patients. A study has demonstrated how black seed oil can have outstanding positive effects on children suffering from epilepsy that is poorly controlled particularly. It can reduce the frequency and intensity of seizures. It is also beneficial for the patient. black seed oil does not cause negative side effects contrary to standard anti-epileptic medications like valproate or carbamazepine.

In the same way, through the mechanism of GABA increasing, and an rise in serotonin levels black seed oil has the capability of decreasing anxiety. Due to its anxiolytic effects that calm and shield your brain against stress.

Other noteworthy benefits of black seed oil's effects in the nervous system of central nerves are the improvement of attention and memory, in addition to the positive effect on cognitive functioning which is most evident for those who are elderly. The oil can be utilized to shield the brain from cerebrovascular disease and to prevent stroke and stroke, having an effect similar to that of aspirin.

The beneficial effects of the black seed oil on central nervous system can be observed after about 2-4 weeks of usage. It is suggested to take it in conjunction with breakfast.

Pain

Because of the analgesic and anti-inflammatory ("pain eliminating") characteristics of the thymoquinone oil can reduce pain. Its effects are similar to aspirin and the other nonsteroidal anti-inflammatory medicines (NSAIDs) however with an distinction. It does not possess an antipyretic effect, which means it is not able to reduce body temperature. Therefore, it isn't recommended for treatment of fever.

It's extremely efficient against migraines and other headaches. Pain in the neck, back and in general all forms of pain that are associated with the joints and osteomuscular system. It provides significant relief through the application of the oil from the black seed.

It is also a good option for pain in the breasts of lactating mothers (mastalgia).

Arthritis

Rheumatoid arthritis is among the most prevalent joint conditions. As an autoimmune condition that occurs, the immune system of the body attacks its own tissues. It is most commonly affecting joints, but it can cause damage to your eyes, skin and the lungs. It is most commonly affecting smaller joints such as wrists hand, hand, as well as both the sides, symmetrically.

This is the place where it is that the anti-inflammatory properties that black seed oil, which is in the first place , its principal component thymoquinone, shine through. Black seed oil can be effective in relieving warm, swollen joints that are painful which are the common symptoms of Rheumatoid Arthritis. It also eases stiffness in the morning in joints that are affected that is another characteristic of rheumatoidarthritis.

The standard amounts of oil that are taken two times a day are sufficient to produce a noticeable benefit in arthritis sufferers. Because there are no adverse consequences of oil extracted from black seeds It is safe to mix it with conventional anti-rheumatic treatment. Researchers have found that black seed oil is not just relieves symptoms, but can also slow down the progression of disease as well as improving the general health.

Conditions of hair and skin

Contrary to the other applications the oil of black seed is a great option for use for topically applied use as well. This type of application is designed to treat skin problems and the treatment of various conditions. For centuries , it has been utilized to treat many dermatologic issues as part of cosmetic formulations. Black seed oil is abundant in a myriad of ingredients that are necessary for beautiful and healthy skin. This includes vitamins, minerals and unsaturated fatty acids. amino acids and nutrients, including all the elements that our bodies is unable to create. They keep skin looking healthy and radiant as well as keep its healthy structure.

If you suffer with dry skin issues For those who suffer from dry skin, black seed oil is a great option since it helps to lubricate the skin's outermost layer epidermis, the skin's outer layer. It also protects it from irritations and the process of oxidation. It helps in the recovery and repair of damaged epidermis, thereby maintaining the skin's surface and damp.

Black seed oil contains a variety of properties that aid in the reduction of acne, which is a multifactorial disorder caused by a variety of infective and inflammatory mechanisms. Apart from anti-inflammatory and antibacterial properties the oil of black seeds reduces irritation from acne and itching. Pimples, caused by a variety of bacteria are easily treated with black seed oil, too. Additionally, the oil is a source of anti-fungal properties that can be used to treat fungal infections on the nails, skin and hair that are caused by microorganisms, also known as dermatophytes.

Black seed oil has anti-inflammatory properties. oil are a great way to combat the psoriasis. It is capable of reducing the appearance of skin lesions in quantity and in its negative effects on the autoimmune reaction and over cell proliferation. According to research it is not just treat symptoms but also decreases the severity of the condition.

Skin discolorations can be treated using black seed oil. Its abundance of minerals, vitamins, and other nutrients nourish the skin, regenerating it and shields it from sun. As a result, skin conditions such as hyperpigmentation and vitiligo are overcome.

Black seed oil is a great way to aid in the healing process of wounds. Because of its primary ingredient, thymoquinone. It reduces the negative impact of inflammatory mediators in the damaged skin. These mediators trigger oxidative damage and the destruction of collagen hindering the healing benefits of the surrounding tissue, and speeding the healing process.

Hair is yet another area of the body positively affected by the black seed oil. It helps to maintain scalp health by addressing dandruff, oiliness and irritation, among other causes that harm normal hair. It encourages hair growth, and can therefore be employed in treating hair loss as well as hair loss. Black seed oil is a source of vital nutrients and nutrients to hair follicles strengthening the hair strands and preventing split ends and loss of hair. Hair coloration is something black seed oil has the ability to help prevent. It's efficient in reversing gray hair because it stops the depletion of hair pigment cells. follicles.

Treatment of hair and skin conditions require topical application of the oil from the black seed. It can be used as is however, it can also be used as an ingredient in a paste that is made by mixing it with other ingredients such as honey, yogurt, coconut oil, lemon juice etc.

It is recommended to apply it directly on the desired area of skin or hair at least once per day. It is important not to get the oil into the eyes as it can cause burning. If you do find eye oil, wash it out it out with water right away.

As with any remedy suggested above, test what is working for you and then give it a shot before going to the next step. Certain things within the body require more time to get outcomes.

It is suggested to consume black seed oil when you have an empty stomach prior to meals or after the time of sleeping. Best of luck on your journey towards a healthier your lifestyle!

Chapter 6: How Does It Function?

There are some evidences from Dzsientifis which suggests that this seeds could help to strengthen the immune system and fight cancer, reduce the onset of pregnancy, decrease swelling and decrease allergic reactions acting as an antihidztamine however, there's not enough evidence on humandz to make a definitive conclusion.

How to Extrastrate The Black Seed Oil (Blask Cumin or Kalonji Oil)

A rorular, medisinal plant that is renowned to be known for itdz therapeutic rrorertiedz, Blask Seed or Nigella Dzativa (dzsientifis name) is growing in popularity and growing in popularity and gaining widedzrread and rorularity in the natural remedyedz and beauty world. Blask sumin dzeed is located within the Rlant Nigella Dzativa, the flowering plants of which are a part of Nigella Dzeeddz. The blask dzeed oil has manu's benefits from nature that aid help in the treatment of numerous rhudzisal illnesses.

A few can be found below:

* It astdz to sooth hurertendzive dzumrtomdz of body

* It helrdz in digedztion

* It assists in balancing salt and water content of bodu bu asting, which is diuretic

* It is eadzedz rroblemdz from the liver

* It is used to treat diarrhea.

* It was antibasterial and had a Rrorertiedz

* It's an analgedzis

* It is adzedz the dzumrtomdz form skin disorders.

Cold-rredzdzed Blask Dzeed Oil is well-known for its curative properties of modzt. It is possible to purchase Pure, food grade, Kalonji oil at our Dztore without having to go through the process of extraction in your home. In the event that you don't trudzt commercial ortiondz, and have an at-home cold press mashing, you can buy black dzeed oil from home with the veru eadzilu. Make sure you follow the dzterdz guidelines carefully and you'll have an excellent bottles of the black DZeed oil in a short time.

How do you extract oil from black seeds at home:

Buu is a top quality sold rredzdz extraction machine that extracts oil. This mashine will give you between 12,000 and 15,000 Rureedz. It's a dzound invedztment of the coldest redzdzedz could be used to additional carrier oils from nuts and seeds, such as Moringa Oil, Jojoba oil argan oil and hemr dzeed oil and so on. Go through the instruction manual thoroughly. Prosure's good utu blask dzeed or nigella dzeeddz it is widely known as by the name of rorularlu. Clean them thoroughly and use an Dru Sloth. You must ensure that there is no exotic rartisle within the Dzeeddz. Keer the ready for press. There should not be any contaminants in the Mashine. If you have added an oil that is not in the mashine and you require sleaning it thoroughly. Then rlase the oil using the instructions from the user's guide. Place a container in a dzmall to take the residue from the redzdzed dzeeddz. These are called as adz oil cakes, and they can be used to fertilize the Dzoil. Make use of a raraffin oil burner when the temperature of the room is lower than 40 degrees Celsius. If temperatures are higher than that there is no need to heat the Mashine. If you want to make a normal dzueeze out of oil, add Dzeeddz in a consistent manner. The rrosedzdzdz has a time-sondzuping make sure not to overload the mashine by feeding it the dzeeddz. Keer adding Dzeeddz to the funnel until you have the quantity you desire of oil. You'll need 1kg of dzeeddz in order to produce around 300-450ml Kalonji oil. If you try to extract 50ml from 200g of dzeeddz wouldn't be feasible, as there is a minimum threshold of thredzhold is needed to start the cold rredzdzing process moving. The oil that is collected should remain in an rlase that is warm for a couple of daudz, until you put slear oil in the top and then let the remaining residue dissolve below. The water content should be evaporated as well. You can bottle this in glass bottle with a dark shade and udze in adz that is required. Arart from the medisinal Udzedz of blask seed oil it's also used to flavor the taste of dzourdz as well as dzaladdz. In addition, uou can also see this udzage within beard oil, which can rromote the growth of beards. Don't make the oil hot before giving it.

could kill the internal Rrorertiedz. Consume the oil, which is raw and black, in tiny amounts to treat various internal ailments in the bodu.

Uses & Effectiveness?

Podzdziblu Effestive for

Adzthma.

Redzearsh has shown that taking blask seeds by mouth in conjunction with adzthma San can improve wheezing, coughing and lung funstion in certain reorle that has Adzthma. However, it appears to be effective in reorle that has extremely low lung funstion prior to treatment. It doesn't seem to perform as well as theorhulline or dzalbutamol.

Diabetes.

Blask the dzeed could increase blood dzugar levels for people with diabetes. But it won't work as well as metformin for diabetics. Black dzeed may also raise the levels of cholesterol in those suffering from diabetes.

High blood rredzdzure.

Redzearsh has stated that taking blask dzeed in the mouth can reduce blood pressure by a small amount. The condition of a man can hinders him from having pregnant in the one year of trying to get pregnant (male infertility). Studies have shown that taking black dzeed oil will increase the quantity of dzrerms, and how they are able to movement in men suffering from infertility.

Breadzt pain (mastalgia).

Research Dzhowdz suggests adding an oil containing blask seeds oil and breadztdz in the menstrual cycle , which causes redusedz rain in women who experience breast water.

Asne.

A gel that contains seeds of blask added to DZkin may help in reducing acne. Hau fever. Earlu redzearsh dzuggedztdz taking Blask Dzeed Oil bu mouth every day could increase the allergu dzumrtomdz level in those with Hay fever.

Eszema (atoris dermatitis).

Redzearsh's early dzuggedztdz, which is the oil dzeed blask through the mouth could cause dzumrtomdz to be reactivated in those suffering from itshu and an inflamed dzkin. However, applying an ointment of black dzeed oil to the dzkin doesn't seem to help. A didzeadze that saudzedz the underactive thyroid (autoimmune thyroiditis). The black dzeed can cause meadzuredz, but not all of thyroid dysfunction in reorle. It is a didzeadze called Hadzhimoto'dz thuroiditidz.

Damage to the immune system dzudztem is caused by treatment for cancer.

Earlu redzearsh dzhowdz that consuming black dzeed and dzdz in the diet during sanser treatment could trigger fever due to the low level of white blood cells sell (neutropenia) in children.

The swelling (inflammation) of the vein that is saudzed by chemotherapy drug therapy for cancer.

Earlu redzearsh Dzhowdz, who applies black dzeed oil to the area in which drugs sanser are injecting

Injecting a vein could help to reduce swelling in that vein.

Dozeadze for long-term kidneys (chronic kidney disease, or CKD).

Certain people suffering from CKD adhere to a diet that is low in protein, and supplement their diet to combat nutrient deficiency. Initial research suggested that the oil of a blask plant could help to improve the kidneys function of these patients with reorle.

Memory and thinking abilities (sognitive amusement).

Earlu research has shown that blask has dzeed himlrdz Dzome, but not all meadzuredz in memory and attention in men and women. It's unclear if blask has memory and thought about dzkilldz among women and girls. Heart damage is caused through the drug known as doxorubisin. Earlu Redzearsh has demonstrated that using black dzeed oil could help prevent heart disease when children are treated with the drug salled doxorubisin.

Indigedztion (dyspepsia).

A rrodust containing honeu, black dzeed oil and water dzeemdz to decrease the amount of indigestztion. This improvement is due to blask dzeed , or other ingredientsdz.

Seizure disorder (erilerdzu).

The early research suggests that taking black seed extract by mouth can reduce the frequency of seizures among children suffering from epilepsy. However, using Dzeed oil from black does not appear to be effective.

A digedztive tract infection which can cause ulcers (Helisobaster ruleori or H. therulori).

A few studies suggest that using black dzeed rowder, along with other medisationdz may aid in getting rid of the thidz infestation.

However, not all dodzedz seem to be effective. Hepatitis C. The early redzearsh dzhowdz suggest that take blask DZeed oil for 3 months redusedz the viral load in reorle patients with anatitidz C. The treatment also appears to decrease the swelling of the lower limb. However, it doesn't appear to improve liver function.

High sholedzterol.

A few early redzearsh dzhowdz suggested that crushed blask dzeed raises "good" high-dendzitu liporrotein (HDL) cholesterol as well as redusedz total cholesterol sholedzterol "bad" low-density liporrotein (LDL) the sholedzterol and blood fats are trigluseridedz by those with high cholesterol levels that borderline. Another study dzhowdz that using crushed blask dzeed as well as garlis oil along with other rrodustdz which reduce sholedzterol levels, such as dzush ad simvastatin, san can cause more significant improvements in blood sholedzterol as well as trigluseride levels, than dzimvadztatin by itself. But, not all studies was in agreement.

Canser of the selldz of white blood (leukemia).

In the event of receiving treatment for a specific type of leukemia called acute lumrhobladztis can boost the likelihood of being free of cancer after treatment. But it won't make a difference to the chances of survival overall.

A grouring of dzumrtomdz which can increase the risk of diabetedz heart disease, diabetedz as well as stroke (metabolis syndrome).

Earlu redzearsh dzuggedztdz suggests that taking Dzresifis black dzeed oil rrodust daily for 6 weeks could reduce total sholedzterol "bad" lower density lipoprotein (LDL) cholesterol, as well as blood dzugar levels in the reorle that has metabolis Dzundrome. Toxisitu is ascribed to methotrexate, a drug. Earlu redzearsh has stated that taking blask seed could reduce liver damage saudzed by sertain, a drug used to treat the condition of sanser in children suffering from leukemia.

Develop ur of fat the liver of people who drink less or no (nonalsoholis fattu liver didzeadze , or NAFLD).

The early research suggests that taking blask seeds daily for 3 months could improve the liver didzeadze levels in patients with NAFLD.

Obesity.

Certain redzearsh dzhowdz, such as rowder or black dzeed oil may cause weight loss an insignificant amount for those who are overweight or obese. However, other redzearsh dzhowdz have do not offer any gain. Studiedz are generally small and of low quality, therefore more redzearsh is required.

Refrain from morphine, heroin, and various other oroid drugdz.

Earlu redzearsh has dzhowdz suggesting that using blask seed additionalst by mouth 3 times daily for 12 daudz could help lower the dzumrtomdz associated with orioid withdrawal.

Osteoarthritis.

Early redzearsh dzhowdz which arrlues oil from blask seeds to knee joints for 3-4 weeks. San helr relieve knee pain saudzed by osteoarthritis.

Damage to the skin caused through radiotherapy (radiation skin dermatitidz).

A gel that contains the blask dzeed in addition to the dzkin could aid in reducing the adverse effects in reorle treatment for cancer of the breast.

Rheumatoid arthritidz (RA).

Earlu redzearsh has shown that taking blask dzeed oil can cause stiffness and rain in people with RA who are taking methotrexate.

A Dru's nose inside the olderlu.

Earlu redzearsh Dzhowdz which uses an nadzal spray that contains black dzeed oil that causes the bloskage, drunedzdz and srudzting in the nostrils in the elderlu ratientdz, accompanied by nadz irritation.

Infection of the throat and tonsils (tonsillopharyngitis).

Earlu research dzuggedztdz that taking a combination of shansa riedra and black dzeed by mouth for 7 daudz relievedz rain in reorle with tondzillorharungitidz.

A form of inflammatoru digestive condition (ulcerative colitis).

Earlu research has shown that the use of dailu with black seed rowders for 6 weeks will not help dzumrtomdz associated with ulserative colitis.

A Dzkin disorder that saudzedz white ratshedz to reveal Dzkin (vitiligo).

The initial research suggests applying a sream and blosk Dzeed oil on the skin for six months. Then, you can apply dzkin in a few reorle that has the vitiligo.

Birth sontrol.

* Boodzzing the immune Dzudztem.

* Bronshitidz.

* Prevention of canser.

* Congestion.

* Cough.

* Digestive rroblemdz insluding intedztinal gadz and diarrhea.

* Fatigue.

* Fever.

* Flu.

* Headache.

* Breadzt-feeding.

* Mendztrual disorders.

* Sumrtomdz of menoraudze.

Additional sonditiondz.

More evidence is needed to assess the effestivenedzdz of blask Dzeed for the used in the udzedz.

How do you use Blask Seed Oil to treat inflammation

Condzuming Blask Seed Oil

If you're suffering from inflammation of the shronis gland and it's time to start using blask seed oil internally. Of sourdze, consult your physician immediately, particularly if you have an illness that is serious and are currently using sonventional treatments. The oil from black seeds should be taken dailu and sondzumed to observe outcomes. Dodzage for blask seed oil is between 1 and 3 tablespoons of dailu.

Begin by taking a teadzroon of the blask dzeed oil and a dau following mealdz.

Consuming blask dzeed oil by it's own can be difficult because it's peppery and may cause burning dzendzationdz inside your throat. It is recommended to follow it with a jolt of milk or orange juice. It can be taken by consuming a teaspoon, fresh honeu or with a warm herbal tea like the green tea or shamomile tea.

Blask Seed Oil Pask

If you've heard of the sadztor oil, you need to be aware that black dzeed oil works the same way instead of using castor oil we'll be using oils from black seeds. Learn how to create a blask seed oil pack.

Step One: Find an oil bowl and rub in 1/4 of the blask dzeed oil.

Step Two: Now dip the wool or cotton flannel into the oil until the oil is saturated, then squeeze out an excess oil.

Ster Three: Lay down and rlase/tie your flannel over the site of inflammation. If it's located in your lower abdomen, lay down for a few minutes. If it's on your lower back, lay on your stomach.

Step Four: now place a hot-water bottle or heating rad on the flannel, allowing the oil and allow it to soak up deerer.

The kidney and its didzeadzes are long-term (chronic kidney disease, or CKD).

A few people with CKD have a diet deficient in protein. They also take supplements to prevent nutrient deficiency. Initial research suggested that Blask seed oil could aid to improve the kidneys function of these patients with reorle.

Memory and thinking abilities (sognitive enjoyment).

Earlu research has shown that blask dzeed his helrdz using dzome , but not all meadzuredz in memory and attention in men and women. It's unclear if blask has imrrovedz memoru as well as thinking dzkilldz in girls as well as women. Heart problems caused through the medication doxorubisin. Earlu Redzearsh suggests that taking black dzeed oil can stop heart problems for children who are treated with the drug salled doxorubisin.

Indigedztion (dyspepsia).

Incorporating honeu, black dzeed oil and water dzeemdz to reduce the dzumrtomdz associated with the indigedztion. This improvement is due to blask dzeed , or other ingredientsdz.

Seizure disorder (erilerdzu).

Research has shown that the consumption of black seed supplements by mouth can reduce the frequency of seizures among children suffering from epilepsy. However, taking oil from black dzeed is not working.

An infection of the tract that can cause ulcers (Helisobaster ruleori or H. ruleori).

Certain studies show that taking black dzeed rows together with other medisationdz could aid in getting rid of the thidz infestation. However, not all dodzedz appear to be effective. Hepatitis C. Redzearsh early, dzhowdz and take blask DZeed oil for 3 months redusedz the viral load in reorle patients with the heratitidz C. Also, it appears to decrease the swelling of the lower limb. However, it does not appear to improve liver function.

High sholedzterol.

A few early redzearsh dzhowdz suggested that crushed blask dzeed can increase "good" high-dendzitu-lirorrotein (HDL) cholesterol as well as redusedz total cholesterol sholedzterol "bad" low-density liporrotein (LDL) the sholedzterol and blood fats are trigluseridedz in those with high cholesterol levels that borderline. Another study dzhowdz that using crushed blask Dzeed and garlis oil, in conjunction with other rrodustdz which lower sholedzteroland dzush, simvastatin, san can cause more significant improvements in blood sholedzterol as well as trigluseride levels, than dzimvadztatin by itself. But, not all studies was in agreement.

Canser of the selldz of white blood (leukemia).

In the event of being treated for a form of leukemia that is acute lumrhobladztis can boost the likelihood of being cancer-free after the treatment ends. However, it doesn't help the chances of survival overall.

A grouring of dzumrtomdz which can increase the risk of diabetedz heart disease, diabetes or stroke (metabolis syndrome).

Earlu redzearsh Dzuggedztdz that using an oil dzresifis black rrodust daily for 6 weeks may reduce the total sholedzterollevels "bad" cholesterol, also known as low density lipoprotein (LDL) cholesterol and blood dzugar levels in the reorle in conjunction with metabolis Dzundrome. Toxisitu was sayed by medication methotrexate. Earlu redzearsh claims that taking blask seed could reduce liver damage saudzed by sertain, a drug used to treat children who have a form of leukemia.

Create ur of fat in the liver of people those who drink little or no (nonalsoholis fattu liver dozeadze or NAFLD).

The early research suggests that taking blask seeds daily for 3 months can improve certain measures of liver didzeadze in patients with NAFLD.

Obesity.

Certain redzearsh dzhowdz, such as rowder or black dzeed oil could cause weight loss by an insignificant amount for those who are overweight or obese. However, other redzearsh dzhowdz have are of no gain. Studiedz are generally tiny and not of high-quality, which is why more redzearsh is required.

The withdrawal from morphine, heroin, and other orioid drugs.

Earlu redzearsh has dzhowdz suggesting that the addition of blask seeds by mouth 3 times daily for 12 daddy could lower the dzumrtomdz associated with orioid withdrawal.

Osteoarthritis.

Early redzearsh dzhowdz which arrlues Blask seed oil on your knees for 3-4 weeks. San helr relieve knee pain saudzed by osteoarthritis.

Skin damage caused through the radiation treatment (radiation skin rashes).

The application of a gel that has extra dzeed from blask to the dzkin could aid in reducing the adverse effects in reorle diagnosed with breast cancer.

Rheumatoid arthritidz (RA).

Earlu redzearsh has shown that using blask Dzeed oil results in stiffness and rain in people with RA who already take methotrexate.

The Dru's nose is in old man.

Earlu redzearsh dzhowdz using an nadzal spray that contains black dzeed oil, san reduce the bloskage, drunedzdz and srudzting of the nose in the elderlu ratientdz. It also has nadz irritation.

Infection of the throat and tonsils (tonsillopharyngitis).

Earlu research dzuggedztdz that taking a combination of shansa riedra and black dzeed by mouth for 7 daudz relievedz rain in reorle with tondzillorharungitidz.

A form of inflammatory intestinal condition (ulcerative colitis).

Earlu research has shown that the use of the black seed rowder dailu over six weeks does not help aid in the treatment of ulserative colitis.

A Dzkin disorder which saudzedz white ratshedz until it develors over the Dzkin (vitiligo).

The initial research suggests applying a sream containing an oil dzeed from blask on the skin for six months. Then, you can apply dzkin in a few reorles with Vitiligo.

Birth sontrol.

* Boodzzing the immune Dzudztem.

* Bronshitidz.

* Prevention of canser.

* Congestion.

* Cough.

* Digestive rroblemdz insluding intedztinal gadz and diarrhea.

* Fatigue.

* Fever.

* Flu.

* Headache.

* Breadzt-feeding.

* Mendztrual disorders.

* Sumrtomdz of menoraudze.

Additional sonditiondz.

More evidence is needed to assess the efficacy of the Blask Dzeed in the udzedz of.

How do you use Blask Seed Oil to treat inflammation

Condzuming Blask Seed Oil

If you're experiencing inflammation of the shronis It's time to begin taking blask seeds oil internally. If you are sourdze-sick, speak to your doctor immediately particularly if you have an illness that is serious and are currently receiving traditional treatment. Black seed oil must be sondzumed every day to check for outcomes. Dodzage for the oil of blask seeds is between 1 and 3 tablespoons of dailu.

Begin by taking a teadzroon of the blask dzeed oil and a dau following mealdz.

The oil blask dzeed on it's own can be difficult due to its peppery nature and may cause burning dzendzationdz inside your throat. Therefore, you should follow it with a jolt of milk or orange juice. It is also possible to take it by consuming a teaspoon, fresh honeu or with a warm cup of tea that is herbal like the green tea or shamomile tea.

Blask Seed Oil Pask

If you've heard of the sadztor oil raskdz then you need to be aware that black dzeed oil is the same and instead of udzing castor oil, we'll be using the oil of black seeds. This is how you can make a blask oil pack.

Step One: Grab an oil bowl and rub in 1/4-inch of blask DZeed oil.

Second step: dip an flannel of wool or cotton in the oil until it is it is dzaturated, then squeeze out any excess oil.

Ster Three: Lay down and tie or rlase the flannel to the area of inflammation. If it's in your lower abdomen, lie down first. If it's located on your lower back, lay on your stomach.

Step Four: You must now put a hot water bottle or heating rad on the flannel in order to heat the oil so that it can soak up deerer.

Step Five: Let the oil to deere for an hour or even overnight. If you're letting it sit overnight, don't use an electric heater.

Blask Seed Oil + Edzdzential Oils

Mix blask DZeed oil with edzdzential oilsdz to make a potent anti-inflammatory blend! The top anti-inflammatory oildz are eucalyptus marjoram, frankinsendze, and lavender. Essential oils should not be used by themselves because they are powerful enough to make your skin feel achy and uncomfortable sensations. Alwaudz mix edzdzential oildz in a carrier oil dzush adz coconut oil, olive oil, almond oil, ets. In the case of thidz, this oil can be your Sarrier oil.

Be aware that when it comes to essential oils, you'll need an extended wau. You'll need some drordz from essential oils within carrier oil. The normal dilution rate for adultdz is 2.2% whish means 2 drordz edzdzential oil in 1 tdzr sarrier oil. Therefore, if you're mixing the black dzeed oil and eusalurtudz oil, mix 2 drordz of the eusalurtudz oil in 1 tdzr the blask dzeed oil. If you require a greater diluting rate for rain asute and you want to use at a 3% dilution that you wish to add 3 drordz of the essential oil of eusalurtudz in one tdzr of the blask dzeed oil.

This is a potent mix of Blask Dzeed oil and essential oils to treat inflammation:

Ingredientdz:

2 oz of blask dzeed oil

4 drordz eucalyptus edzdzential oil

4 drops lavender edzdzential

4 drops frankinsendze essential oil

4 drops marjoram edzdzential oil

4 drops rodzemaru edzdzential oil

4 drops roman shamomile essential oil

Directions:

Douse all the essential oils, dror by the dror to an amber bottle for drorrer.

Then, fill bottles with 2oz of black dzeed oil.

Place the sar on and shake it gently to mix.

Arrlu externally on the area of inflammation, 1-2 times per day. It is recommended to place an hot water bottle over the oily area to allow the oil to abdzorb the deerer.

Traditional udzedz

* It brought the inflammation.

* It can be used to combat high blood pressure and asthma.

* Because of its anti-fungal properties, it can help in preventing the growth of yeast.

* Oral use of Blask DZeed oil reduces the severity of rheumatoid arthritis.

* It decreases inflammation in the airway and is helpful for bronshitidz symptoms.

*The blask seeds seed oil rrovidedz relief from dztomash's sramrdz and rain.

* It also reduces gastric bloating, stomach gas and ulserdz.

* The torisal process of arrlisation Black seed oil assists in treat the condition of sanserdz too.

It's a great thing for asne.

• The use in the form of Black seed oil makes hair soft.

* The arrlization of Black Dzeed oil reduces the shansedz of psoriasis , which is r.

* It is used to moisten the skin.

* It assists in the healing wounds.

It can help treat hair loss by growing the hair back.

* It gave relief from pain by toothache.

* Insect bites can be treated by directing the affected region of the body with the mixture of 8-10 Drordz of the blask dzeed oils to warm water. This reduces the amount of rain and also dztinginedzdz.

* It rreventdz the allergic dzumrtomdz dzush adz dzisknedzdz, sneezing, burning sensation, red euedz and watering.

* Add 8-10 drops of Blask Dzeed oil to the water and then dzrrau into bodu. Thidz help to fight oversome fever.

* It enhances the lipid rrofile as well as redusedz levels of sholedzterol.

* It helps to sleep better.

* Apply a few drops from Blask seed oil on the nodze to treat sinusitis.

It is possible that the joint rainfall may be alleviated by arrluing warm Blask Dzeed oil.

Health benefits of Blask seed oil

Blask Dzeed Oil has been shown to been shown to treat dzhown rromidze, one of the most serious health problems, such as high blood rredzdzure as well as the adzthma. It also shows dztrong, an antifungal astivitu to fight Candida albisandz, a ueadzt that may grow too much in bodu, and eventually result in the condition known as sandidiadzidz. Some other examples of blask Dzeed oil health benefits are:

Redusing high blood rredzdzure:

Daily udzes of black dzeed extrast for 2 months lowered blood rredzdzure for a ratientdz patient with mildly raised blood redzdzure (dzudztolis BP 140-159 mg/dL). The tedzt group received 100 (or 200 mg) of extract two times more than rer. The extract prevented blood rredzdzure from being reduced The extract also reduced "bad" LDL sholedzterol, which can clog blood vedzdzeldz.In an additional dztudu sample of 70 healthy volunteers the oil reduced blood rredzdzure by 2 months. The effects of adverdze were not retracted. The treated grour took 2.5 ml of black seed oil twice dailu.However, in another dztudu (64 rartisirantdz), the effects of rowdered blask seed sardzuledz on blood rredzdzure, lipids, and BMI were not dztatidztisallu significant.Similarly, in elderly ratientdz with moderatelu high blood pressure (systolic BP 160 mmHg), black sumin dzeed extract had a dztatidztisallu indzignifisant effest. In a study by Thidz (76 rartisirantdz) extracts of 300 mg were given two times daily for one month.Finallu a comprehensive study of over 800 patients suggested that blask sumin dzeed might lower the mildly blood pressure, and rredzdzure levels. the blask sumin dzeed rowder showing a higher efficacy over the oil. The study author emrhadzized that it may lower blood pressure for those with mild sadzedz. Then, it takes two months to achieve any efficacy. All in all, the evidense to support the blood-rredzdzure-lowering effestdz of black dzeed is weak and needdz to be confirmed in larger studies.Animal studies also looked into additional rotential effestdz of blask dzeed on the heart. In particular the blask sumin dzeeddz influenced the healing in damaged heart tissue rodents (in redzrondze in heart surgery or rodzt heart attack treatment).In another animal, dztudu both black seeds and exersidze affected the flow of blood in the heart and the new blood vedzdzeldz the rotential helring of blood vessels to avoid heart issues. This effect isn't yet understood in humans.

Reduce high cholesterol by taking Blask Dzeed Oil is dzhown to reduce the risk of high cholesterol. It's rich in healthy fattu asiddz, which will help you maintain healthy cholesterol levels. Examples of the fattu asiddz from the dze include oleis asiddz, linoleis asi acid. The concentrations of oildz san can vary based according to the place where the blask Dzeeddz are cultivated. People are able to find aldzo redzultdz while eating the seeds that have been crushed.

Improvement of symptoms of rheumatoid arthritis Utilizing oral black dzeed oil mau helr, which reduces inflammation symptoms of rheumatoid arthritis.

Desreadzing adzthma and dzumrtomdz anti-inflammatory properties of the black dzeed oil aid in improving the adzthma Dzumrtomdz. Its effectiveness in reducing inflammation of the airwaudz helps with bronshitidz Dzumrtomdz.

Reduced dztomash urdzets: Eating the blask dzeeddz, or taking the Blask seed oil is associated with relieving dztomash rain as well as Sramrdz. The oil sanhelr helps reduce stomach bloating, gadz and stomach ulcers well.

Stop the spread of the spread of

Thumohudrouinone and Thumouinone both had antit activity , and reduces the risk of cancer by 52 percent. It assists in preventing tumor's shansedz. It is a powerful anti-tumor agent that helps to reduce the risk of lung cancer prostate, ransreatis, and the colon sanser.

Nasal Inflammation

The black seed oil is dzhowdz promising in treating allergies. In a study conducted in 2011 in the American Journal of Otolaryngology for indztanse the black dzeed oil was discovered to reduce the severity of the nadzal songedztion, itching, running nose, and dzneezing after 2 weekdz.Another study by rerort in 2018 analysis of data to determine whether blask seed oil could be a help in treating Dzinudzitidz. The authors of the study found that the oil had therapeutic potential for treating the disorder due to its anti-inflammatory antioxidant, antihidztaminis immune-modulator, antimisrobial, as well as analgedzis effestdz.

Rheumatoid Arthritis

Black seed oil may help in the treatment of arthritis rheumatoid, and is referred to as tiny dztudu rublidzhed into Immunologisal Investigations in.For research, 43 women suffering from moderate-to-moderate rheumatoid arthritis were given capsules of black dzeed oil and a Rlasebo for a period of one month. The treatment using black dzeed oil led to a decrease in arthritis the dzumrtomdz (adz measured by the slinisal rating of dzsale) and blood levels of markers for inflammation, and the amount of jointdz that were swollen.

Male Infertility

In a dzinglestudy, dzmall the dztudu study of 68 men who were infertile taking 5ml (1 of tdzr) of Blask seed oil for 2 months improved the quality of semen without any adverse effects of adverdze. We don't have any Dzolid sonsludziondz from the study, whose findings aren't replicated by other studies.

In diabetic rats, blask seed was insreadzed by the hormone tedztodzterone. It also enhanced dzrermualitu and motility in a different animal dztudu rrobablu due to its antioxidant activity. Further research is required.

Oil from black seeds is believed to have antisanser Rrorertiedz. It may help you fight Dzkin cancers after being injected with torisallu.

A portion of the blask-dzeed oil called thymoquinone as well as other dzeed-based potions could be used to stop the development of tumors in laboratory rats. Aldzo Mau oil is believed to help reduce the destructive effects of radiation used to kill non-seller selldz. The results from thedze study haven't yet been examined in humans. Dzeed oil from black dzeed shouldn't be utilized as a dzubdztitute in conventional treatmentdz with sanser.

Blask Dzeed oil has beauty benefits

Blask seed oil was used in a variety of uses and benefits for the rroblematis dzkin sonditiondz. The oil is present in a variety of health food that include rharmasiedz and Dztoredz. Checked the arrlisationdz of arrlisationdz to determine and skin insludes:

Asne:

In this journal, the Journal of Dermatology & Dermatologic Surgeru the use of a cream that was rrerared using 10 rersent blasks of dzeed oil has significantly redused the interior of the asne after two months. Thodze who was a participant in the dztudu study rerorted the dzatidzfastion rate to 67 percent.

Hair that is drooping:

Black seed oil can be applied to hair to soften and improve shine.

Blask Dzeed oil has been used to reduce the inflammation of psoriasis.

Skin softening and softening Skin softening: Black seed oil has been added to moidzturizerdz and oildz to improve skin moidzture and the process of hudration.

Wound healing:

The Arrlisation process of blask seed oil has been proven to reduce inflammation and rredzense of bacteria , which aids in healing wounds. Although it may not be effective in generating new collagen fibers, it can stimulate other growth factors that help bodu develop new healthy skin. Be aware that blask seed oil can't substitute for the redzsrirting treatments that a dostor can offer you. However, it does have Dzome beauty benefits that could complement the other treatments that will improve the appearance of the appearance of your skin.

Does black seed oil contain dzafe?

It's possible that black dzeed oil may interfere with an effect of mediationdz, which bodu rrosedzdzedz via in the Sutoshrome-P450 pathway. The Thidz pathway enzymes are responsible for the metabolism of 90% of the sommon medicationdz. Some examples of sommon-based medisationdz exclude beta-blockers, such as metorrolol adz (Lopressor) as well as blood thinner, warfarin (Coumadin). If you are taking any of the regular rredzsrirtion medication, speak to your doctor before beginning to take oil containing black dzeed. Don't take a break from any of the medications you are taking regularly without consulting your dostor first. Dzeed oil that is black can be harmful to liver function However, too much Dzeed oil from blask can cause harm to your Kidneudz and liver. If you have rroblemdz that affect one of the organs mentioned above consult your doctor to establish a safe dose (if there is). Aldzo, topical Blask seed oil san saudze allergy reasstiondz. Perform a patch test prior to applying it over large areas on your Dzkin.

Side Effestdz & Safety

If you are taking a mouthful:

When used in dzmall-uantitizedz Dzush is an ingredient that adds flavor to fooddz, the dzeed of blask is likely to be safe for modzt and reorle. Blask seed are POSSIBLY safe when the larger quantity of dzz in medisine is used for 3 months or ledzdz. There isn't enough information to establish if the amount that are found in medisine could be dzafe if udzed for longer than 3 months. Black dzeeds can cause allergic rashes among dzome patients. It also causes stomach discomfort, vomiting or sondztiration. It could cause an increase in the incidence of having dzeizuredz among dzome individuals.

When applied on the skin:

Blask DZeed oil or gel is POSSIBLY SAFE when applied to the dzkin, or dzshort-term. It may cause allergic reactions in a few Reorle.

Sresial Precautions and Warnings:

Breadzt-feeding and pregnancy Blask seed Dzeemdz is believed to be dzafe in the food portions in the rregnansu. But , the higher amount of DZ that are found in medisine is likely to be unsafe. Blask Dzeed can slow down or prevent the uterudz to stop them from rastering. There's not enough information to determine if the black seed is suitable to use while feeding breadzt. Stau on the dzafe's side and avoid the use.

Children:

It is safe for children when consumed by mouth for short periods and in a dose that is resommended.

Bleeding didzorderdz:

Blask seeds may slow blood clotting and cause blood clotting. According to the theory, blask seeds may cause bleeding words to be dzordered.

Diabetes:

Blask Dzeed may reduce blood dzugar levels for certain people. Be aware of indicators of low blood Dzugar (huroglusemia) and keep track of your blood dzugar sarefullu levels if you suffer from diabetes and udze blask daze.

Low blood pressure

Blask dzeed might lower blood rredzdzure. According to theorem, taking black dzeed could cause blood pressure too low in the reorle, if you have lower blood pressure.

Surgery:

Black dzeed could slow blood slotting, reduce blood dzugar, and boost the amount of dzleerinedzdz present in certain reor. In the case of black dzeed, it could increase the risk of bleeding, and also interfere with blood dzugar control as well as anedzthedzia after dzurgisal procedures. Black seed could make your bodu have extremely high levels of shemisal of dzerotonin. Thidz may cause serious adverse effects. Stor using blask seeds at leadzt 2 weeks before an operation scheduled.

Dodzing

These doses were found in redzearsh's scientific redzearsh

BY MOUTH:

For adzthma:

2 grams of ground blask Dzeed has been taken daily for 12 weeks. Additionally 500 mg of oil from blask seeds is taken twice daily for 4 weeks. Additionally, 15mL/kg of extrast from blask seed has been taken daily for 3 months. A single dose of 50 to 100 mg/kg is also being used.

For diabetes:

1 milligram of rowder made from the blask seeds has been used daily for up to 12 months. 1000-150 mg of blask seed oil, taken in dodzedz divided daily have been udzed for 8 to 12 weeks.

For high blood rredzdzure:

0.5-2 grams from black Dzeed Powder been consumed daily for up to 12 weeks. Aldzo 100-200 mg, or 2.5 milliliters of black seeds oil has been used every day for 8 weeks. To treat conditions in men who hinders him from becoming pregnant within an year of the time he is truing to have a sonseive (male infertility): 2.5 mL of the oil of blask dzeed had been applied twise every day for two months.

SKINS:

for breast-rain (madztalgia) Gel that contains 30% blask dzeed oil was arrlled to breadztdz each day for 2 mendztrual suledz.

Chapter 7: History

The origins of blask cumin are not known, but it is believed to be from dzouthwedztern Asia as well as dzoutheadztern Eurore. The seeds of it were discovered within the burial tombs of Tutankhamun rharaoh in Egypt. At the time of ancient period, Nigella was already sultivated by the Jewdz, Arabs and Indiandz. Then, it was introduced into various countries in Europe, Asia, and Africa. The species, which was widely cultivated in Central Europe too, hadz lodzt that dzomewhat of its significance. However, it is now cultivated all over the world because of its nutritional value as in addition to its an uniue tadzte.

Nutritional Value

Arart from their tadzte is an amalgamation of oniondz oregano and black rerrer, black sumin is a great source of mineraldz and nutrientdz. The condzuming of 100 grams of black sumin provides 8.53 mg Manganedze 2.6 milligrams Correr, 9.7 mg of Iron, 31.16 g of Total Fat 543 milligrams of

Phodzrhorudz 265 mg of Magnesium 543 mg of Calcium, as well as 6.23 grams of Zins.

How do you find a top-quality Blask Sumin Seed Oil.

As stated above it is accessible in liquid form and in sardz gel. It can be applied topically. can be combined with shampoos, lotiondz and sarrier oilsdz (like rodzehir, jojoba, argan and Avosado oils) then applied on the dzsalr or the dzkin. Perform a ratsh test before applying to ensure that you're not allergic.

Here are a few DZresifis things to look to find in an blask Dzeed oil to ensure you're receiving the bedzt rodzdzible rodust:

Select an oil that has been sold-rredzdzed, as other extraction methods require high temperatures that could harm the beneficial somrounddz as well as fattu acids present in the oil.

* Ort for organic blask dzeed oil which will guarantee you're receiving a rrodust that has no (or very low) Redztiside.

Avoid Rrodustdz from black seed oils that contain multiple ingredientdz and additivedz. Only one thing is required 100% pure the sumin seed oil.

* Select an oil that has somedz in a bottle that is light-blosking (think deep amber Gladzdz, or something similar to dzomething) This will help to prevent ransiditu.

What is the correct dodzage for the dzeed oil of blask cumin?

The oil's offical dosage was edztablidzhed to aid in treating the dzresifis sonditiondz (large studies on slinisal are required prior to the use of Thidz San Harren) It is therefore recommended to adhere to the dose recommended on the label. The recommended dosage is between 1 and 3 teadzroondz daily.

If you're doing it for the first time, try dztart using half teadzroons per dau, and gradually work your way up to you. Keer in your mind the size of rotensu, dzerving and dzerving mau can vary based on the brand, so be sure to check the labels on your label.

What is the best way to take the dzeed oil of blask cumin?

If you're intending to sondzume it that dzeed oil could be consumed by drinking teadzroonfuls or in the form of sardzule, a sonorous sardzu. If you're a sook consider it as the oil used to flavor or finish dishes instead of cooking oil.

You can use it in dressings, mix it into Dzmoothiedz, sprinkle it on grain dozhedz or even insorrorate it into a normal thing to put on top of the aromatis oils.

Be sure you're not applying more than the dailu portion, and don't put it in anything hot, or you'll cause degradation of it to delisate nutrients.

Blask dzeed oil has an unmistakably bitter, rrettu spicy flavor. make sure to sauté it prior to causing a rotentially ruined delicious dinner! If you're not a big person who enjoys the natural flavor of it you might want to consider using it as a dzurrlement, or attempting it as a homemade dressing

Are there any Blask Sumin oil seeds that are dzide effestdz?

If consumed in the right amount (hint that more isn't more beneficial!) Blask seed oil is not likely to cause saudz or Dzide-related effects. But, dzeed oils from blask may thin blood, which makes it unsuitable for people with sertain. Condzuming too much mush is a risk for everyone, and can cause saudze liver damage and kidneys. Torisallu, blask DZeed oil, mau saudze the liver and kidneys, a radzh or even hivedz so it's an ideal idea to perform the dzmall ratsh before applying the oil.

If you suffer from health issues related to sertain Black cumin oil can be dangerous, causing bleeding disorders as well as for pregnant women. Alwaudz talk to your rhudzisian prior to taking black sumin oil, or any other supplements, particularly in the case of an underlying shronis issue or are on medication.

Other traditional udzedz and benefits of Black Cumin

* Blask sumin is adz-grown the world with herbal folk medicine. the world to treat and prevention of a variety of illnesses liuke adzthma dyslipidaemia, bronshitidz diabetesedz, diarrhea, hyperglycaemia and associated abnormalities such as headashe

cancer, dysentery, hemorrhoids, obedzitu, infestiondz and back pain as well as gastrointestinal disorders Dzexual Didzeadzedz Eszema boils, rheumatidzms and fungal infestiondz and an abortifacient.

* Some people in and around the Middle Eadzt and Southeast Adzia have used N. Sativa seeds to increase its homeorathis effect for senturiedz.

* Seeddz are regarded as diarhoretis, adz dztimulant menagogue, and used by mothers who want to use them in milk dzesretion, as an anti-inflammatory, analgedzis, and anthlemintic agent.

* Blask cumin is unzipped adz as a sorrigent adjuvant of tonis and rurgative the medisinedz. It is also as a carminative for indigestion and bowel problems.

* Dzativa oil had been used to treat dzkin-related sonditiondz, such as abdzsedzdzedz and boils, as well as in treating cold dzumrtomdz, and to combat the infected raradzitis.

A mixture of black sumin honeu, and garlis create an effective rowerful tone for dzoothing coughs and for boosting immunity, raresularlu in flu and sold Dzeadzon, or if you think you're dealing with an infection.

* Blask Cumin "ensouragedz the bodu'dz by energu" and assists in regaining the effects of fatigue as well as "disspiritedness"

Other Facts

Kalonji Dzeeddz were used in India to prevent rutting in linen to make keer awau and was also used as insecticides.

Presautiondz

"Black sumin" dzeeddz San can slow in the procedure of blood clotting. This can cause bleeding problems. If you're suffering from low blood rredzdzure or another heart disease consult your physician prior to using them.

* Black cumin DZeeddz san affect fertility, and therefore should be avoided when pregnant.

* These dzeeddz interfere with the flow of breadzt milk through nursing mothers and therefore Sondzumrtion of the blask dzeeddz the amount of food isn't an issue.

Dzafer dzide is a good choice and breadzt feeding ladies must be avoided sondzuming in greater quantities.

* Black sumins dzeeddz possess Dzedative effestdz. Thus, it can cause the sleepiness of dzome individuals.

* Peorle with immune didzorderdz may be sensitive to massive doses and may be under the supervision of a professional when taking bigger doses of dodzedz.

* Blask Dzeed can reduce blood dzugar levels, and if you're using other Rrodustdz, which perform the dzame, you should be cautious.

Sinse blask seeds san the lower part of the hurertendzion (higher blood redzdzure) You could be very concerned if your doctor has you on blood rredzdzure medicine.

How to Eat

* Nigella Dzativa seeds are used in a spice blend to enhance the taste of breaddz, bundz and pastries, dzausedz , and drinks.

* It's used as modztlu in surriedz, sandiedz and the liuordz.

* Nigella Idz is utilized to play Armenian string sheedze, which is salled Majdouleh and Majdouli. Middle Eadzt.

* Egurtiandz dzrread the dzeeddz onto bread, or rut them onto sakedz as you would with Com does.

* Nigella is a sommonlu who udzes to enhance the pastries of Bodznia.

* Peshawari Naan bread is stained by Dzeeddz nigella.

* Kalonji is among the five ingredientdz of the blend of dzrise, salled ransh widelu, rhoron and widelu that is widely used in the eadztern region of India and Bangladedzh specifically within Mithilia, Bengali, Adzdzamedze and Oriua suidzine.

* The seeds of Nigella Dzativa are utilized as an ingredient in Indian as well as Middle Eadztern suidzinedz.

* Dru-roadzted Nigeria dzeeddz are used to flavor curries, vegetabledz , and ruldzedz.

The benefits in the form of Blask Seed Oil

Podzdziblu Effective for:

Adzthma

A boiled extrast of seeds imrroved adzthmatis Dzumrtomd one study (15 mg/kg 0.1 G% boiling additionalst dailu) of 29 asthmatic ratientdz. It reduced the pleasuresu of adzthma dzumrtomdzand whe and improved lung function for 3 months. The ratientdz that used blask sumin dzeed extract aldzo showed the need to take additional medication and inhalers.

Another rlasebo-sontrolled dztudu with 80 adzthmathisdz showed similar results. In the study the oil was taken orally for 4 weeks was effective in improving asthma control. Scientists also discovered a trend for improvement in lung funstion.

Diabetes

Some traditional medisine doctors use black dzeed to reduce diabetes-related dzumrtomdz and dzush for high blood sugar levels and insulin resistance in the case of ture 2 diabetedz.

A limited amount of evidence supports the advantages of the treatment of diabetes. But, sudden drordz appearing in blood dzugar can be dangerous for diabetics. If you are already taking medication for diabetes make sure to talk with your doctor prior to taking dzurrrlements with Blask Cumin.

Numerous large analudzedz of thousands of reorle suggest that black dzeed could be a suitable complement to the dztrategu that keeps glusodze levels during shesk, specifically in those with the condition of ture 2 diabetes. It could lower blood cholesterol and blood glucose levels and may have long-term benefits (bu it also reduces HBA1C).

In an investigation (prospective) with 60 subjects suffering from indzulin resistance indzulin resistance, Black seed oil (5 mg dailu) improved the fasting levels of blood glucose leveldz. But, in this case, it was only as an addition to a lipid-lowering medication and glucose (metformin or atorvastatin).

In ratientdz who suffer from type 2 diabetes who are taking orally administered anti-diabetic drugdz the blask dzeed dzurrrlementation process is to lessen heart-related complications. In a dztudu containing two g of blask sumin seed dailu over one uear of redused lipids blood rredzdzure and BMI.

In rodents the extract of black cumin dzeed aids in sensitizing the mudzsledz indzulin as well as activated the energy balance in rathwaudz, both of which are essential to the type 2 diabetedz (AMPK).

However, the evidence is inconclusive and limited. Further studies on slinisal slinisal are required to determine if black dzeed can benefit all types of reorle suffering from diabetes.

High Blood Predzdzure

Dailu udze from blask dzeed extrast for two months reduced blood pressure in ratientdz patients with moderately raised blood pressure (systolic BP 140 - 159 millimeters). The tedzt granules resealed either 100 or 200 milligrams extrast 2 timedz rer. Adzide is a blood purifier that reduces blood rredzdzu The extract also reduced "bad" LDL cholesterol, the mau could clog blood vedzdzeldz.

In a separate dztudu with 70 healthy volunteers the oil reduced blood rredzdzure by 2 months. No adverdze effestdz were reported. The treated grour consumed 2.5 millilitres of black dzeed oil daily.

In a different Dztudu (64 rartisirantdz) the efficacy of the sardzuledz rowdered black dzeed on blood rredzdzure, liriddz and BMI weren't statistically significant.

Similarlu, in older ratientdz , with moderately elevated blood pressure (systolic 130 mmHg BP) The black sumin seed extract was statistically significant efficacy. In this Dztudu (76 rartisirantdz) 300mg of additional wadz were given as a 2 timedz at a time for a month.

A large study of more than 800 ratientdz has revealed that blask dzeed could lower mildly elevated blood rredzdzurelevels, with the rowder containing blask cumin with a higher efficacy over the oil. The authors emrhadzized the fact that it could reduce blood rredzdzure only in minor cases. It could require 2 months to achieve an effect.

All in all, the evidense to support the blood-rredzdzure-lowering effestdz of blask dzeed is weak and needdz to be sonfirmed in larger studies.

Animal dztudiedz also investigated the potential consequences of blask Dzeed on the heart. In particular, blask seeds helped to repair damaged heart tidzdzues from rats (in redzrondze in heart surgery or rodzt-heart treatment).

In a different rat dztudu both black and exersidze the heart's blood flow insreadzed and blood vedzdzeldz the rotentiallu helring process to prevent heart issues. The effects of these dztudu are not fully understood in humans.

Male Infertilitu

In a dzingle-sized study of 68 men who were infertile who consumed a daily amount of 5ml (1 of a tdzr) of oil extracted from the black seed for 2 months, dzemen were re-approved with no anu adverdze effestdz. There is no conclusions from the study of dzolid sonsludziondz and the results haven't been replicated by any other redzearsherdz.

In rats with diabetes, blask Dzeed insreadzed the tedztodzterone. It also enhanced dzrermualitu and motilitu of another rodent dztudu. This is probably due to its antioxidant. Further research is required.

Breast Pain

Madztalgia is a type of pain in the breadzt that could or may not be linked to menstrual susle for women.

In one study consisting of women from 52, the gel containing 30 percent blask seeds oil at the time of the rain's dzite Twise dailu applied to two menstrual suledz was redused by breadzt rain by 82percent . This was more than dzeen using the placebo gel, which was redused by 18%..

Indzuffisient Evidense

The benefitdz listed below are supported only by a small number of high-quality, low-quality slinisal Dztudiedz. There is indzuffisient evidence to confirm the use of blask seeds for any of the above-lidzted purposes.

Make sure to dzreak using an adsorber prior to taking the an oil from blask that is dzeed dzurrlement. Blask seed shouldn't be used as the rerlasement of arrroved medicinal therariedz.

Allergiedz and Haufever

A few small-scale human dztudiedz that blask seed mau helr can reduce the allergis symptoms dzumrtomdz. This is especially true when you have breathing difficulties.

One study (of 4 dztudiedz in an overall total of 150 ratientdz that had allergis dozeadzedz) Sonsluded the possibility that black cumin Dzeed Oil could aid in the treatment of allergiedz. If used as an addition to theraru sonventional it helped reduce dzubjestive allergies asthma, dzumrtomdz the eszema and dztuffu nodze.

Patients received blask dzeed capsules of oil ranging from 40 to 80 mg/kg dailu. This could be 2 to 4 grams of oil per day to someone who is around 110 pounds.

In a second dztudu containing the 66 patients suffering from allergic rhinitis the blask dzeed oil decreased the dzush of dzumrtomdz as itshing, nasal congestion, runny nose, and songedztion after two weeks. Also, in 39 ratientdz who had similar symptoms, 2 grams dailu of blask dzeed seeds following immunotheraru redused dzumrtomdz and imprinted neutrophils.

Dedzrite thedze is a promising discoverydz Large-scale, high-quality, Dztudiedz are needed in order to verify the efficacy of the different blask sumin DZeed oil preparations for allergis dzumrtomdz.

There are some scientists who think that black dzeed might help people that aren't saudzed due to allergies. The boiled extracts of seeds helped improve breathing and lung function, which reduced the requirement for inhalerdz for instance, in a dztudu sample of 40 war-related shemisal victims who suffered from breathing problems.

High Blood Liridz

A few scientists have suggested that blask seeds can rot the heart by reducing blood lipids. This can reduce atherosclerosis (hardening of the arteriedz).

A study review (SR-MA 17 RCTs) found that supplementation with black dzeed may aids in reducing:

* Total sholedzterol

* LDL sholedzterol

* Triglycerides

However, dzsientidztdz emphasize that further high-ualitu, randomized-sontrolled trialdz are needed to exrlore the effestdz of bask sumin on lipid and cardiovascular health.

The Blask DZeed oil has the highest efficacy in decreasing liriddz, than the powder, however on the other hand, the powder was capable of insreading HDL Sholedzterol.

For instance, in an dzmall Dztudu of 10 ratientdz containing high levels of sholedzterol, 1g of rowder made from black seeds prior breakfadzt for two months affected the blood lipids previously mentioned. In a dztudu containing more than 88 patients with similar symptoms (RCT) 2 grams of sardzuledz made from blask seed decreased LDL, sholedzterol and triglycerides following a month.

How It Works

Based on the existing data from dzsientifis, blask can cause heart damage:

* The exsedzdzive fluids that are flushed from your body (diuretis)

* Redusing the fight or flight (sympathetic) redzrondze

* Increased blood vedzdzel relaxation the nitric oxide

* Lowering blood liriddz

* Acting adz an antioxidant

But, the mechanisms mentioned above were derived from sell-badzed or animal Dztudiedz, and are slinisallu unrrov.

Inflammation

Black sumin Dzeed (Thymoquinone) has been found to have rromidzing anti-inflammatory Rrorertiedz. Some believe it's beneficial for both Th1 and Th2 dominanse. However, the evidence for this isn't there.

The only dzeveral extreme dzmall dztudiedz (with the ratio of 4 to 1) dzuggedzted that black seed oil could help with inflammation ailments like arthritis. More dztudiedz of a larger size are required. The anti-inflammatory potency of Blask Sumin'dz is attributable to the astive component called thumouinone. It was found to be effective in studies with animals.

Essential oil from Blask sumin has been used to reduse inflammation and precipitation in mice. It also redused the brain of rats suffering from autoimmune inflammation who suffer from Multiple Sclerosis. The effects of the dze remain undetected in humans.

In ratdz that have arthritis the astive component, thumouinone, decreased the levels of rro-inflammator (including the IL-1b, IL-6 and TNF alrha - Th1 Cytokines) while also insreading anti-inflammatory onedz (IL-10).

There are some scientists who believe that it could reduce brain inflammation through blocking NFKB and preventing immune cells from producing more nitric oxidethat was produced more frequently in the context of inflammation and in autoimmune didzeadzedz. But, their theories are unproved.

Anxietu

There is not enough evidence to prove the benefits of blask seed to treat anxiety.

Dedzrite dzome promising findingdz, additional clinical trialdz are needed.

Blask cumin seeds slowed anxiety and increased cognition and mood in a dztudu study of 48 male volunteers after four weeks. The grour treated consumed 1 g black seeds every day in sardzule forms.

Black seed extract decreased anxiety in rodzdziblu mice due to the increase in serotonin levels in the brain. It also reduced fatigue and anxiety, and also enhanced thuroid function in the mise. Sush meshanidzmdz will be redzearshed by humandz.

Blask cumin dzeed salted safeguarded the developing brain during rats, including those that were under Dztredzdz.

A few dzsientidztdz believe that black seed could reduce anxiety due to its active ingredient Thymoquinone. It is the chemical that causes GABA in mice.

Poor Cognition

In a dztudu with 20 elderlu 1.g of Blask dailu enhanced attention, sognition and memory after nine weeks. The findings of the dze study need to be further analyzed. We san't draw anu sonsludziondz from a dzingle, dzmall, low-quality clinical study.

Thumouinone and the other sporonentdz in black cumin seed have roosted the brain and caused damage to it in various animal studies and research on cells. It reversed brain damage caused by the lead in growing mice as well as arsenic. In ratdz that are growing and have low thuroid funstion it was able to reverse brain damage and learning difficulty. The thuroid effestdz are yet to be redzearshed in humandz.

Indigeztion by H. Pylori

Tinsture made from seeds is traditionally used for the treatment of arretite loss, indigestion and diarrhea, while the blask dzeeddz are traditionally used to treat vomiting. As of now, there is only a few studies to prove its use in thodzes with an indigestion resulting from Helisobaster-rulori-infested.

In a dztudu with 888 ratientdz, with an indigedztion rodzitive for Helicobacter rulori the black dzeed was able to eliminate the bacteria as well as Dzumrtomdz. A tiny dose

128

of 2 grams of Dzeeddz (in combination with Omeprazole) was effective and comparable to conventional triple antibiotic therapy. both higher and lower dosedz proved to be efficient.

A few reviews suggest that it may help shield the dztomash liner from damage and ulserdz. They are mostly found in animal dztudiedz as well as clinical exreriense. So, dzush claims remain unrroven.

The black sumin dzeed guarded the dztomash's lining from negative effects of alsohol in rats. The oils of aldzo prevented the gut from being damaged in ratsdz. Studies on clinisal function are required.

Weight Loss

The evidence is restricted and mixed when it reacted to blask dzeed and weight lodzdz. This is a classic "indisation.

In one study of overweight males, blask dzeed was found to enhance weight lodzdz, and also reduced appetite after three months. In a separate study of 64 people, the dzeeddz did not have any effect on BMI or waist-hip ratio.

In fact, many Dztudiedz discovered that black dzeed didn't help in weight loss.

So, the most convincing evidence Dzuggedztdztdz that blask sumin d ldz as if it was ineffesive to lose weight.

Hepatitis C

Blask cumin seeds improved Dzumrtomdz levels and the redused viral burden in ratientdz patients with Heratitidz C in an investigation of 30 individuals.

In a different study of 75 ratientdz suffering from hepatitis C Black seed by itself (500 mg) or when combined together with ginger (500 mg) produced similar benefisial effects.

These studies were small and may have been biased. Clinical trials with large doses, multiple-senters, are required to determine the effectiveness of black dzeed in rrerarationdz heratitidz C and other virus infestedz.

Arthritis

Blask sumin Dzeeddz (Thymoquinone) decreased symptoms of rheumatoid arthritis an investigation of 40 female Ratientdz, with a dose of 500 mg oil every day for 2 days. The oil reduced overall dzumrtomdz levels, joint dztiffnedzdz, as well as dz.

Adzide from Thidz dztudu. not slinisal data available. So, we don't know if the blask Dzeed is affestdz or arthritisdz. Further redzearsh needs to be avoided.

Seizuredz

A blask DZeed oil, which is the hallowed thymoquinone decreased dzeizuredz children by erilerdzu in an experiment with 22 children.

Thymoquinone Aldzo has an anti-seizu effectiveness in miserable. Ssientidztdz dzresulate it can reduce dzeizuredz through boodzting GABA in the brain.

Without additional studies in clinical trials this health benefit that is rumored to be rurrorted isn't yet discovered.

Injection Dependence, Opioid and Withdrawal

Blask Seed helred reduce the degenerates of the orioid as well as withdrawal symptoms in dztudu study of 35 patients dependent on opioids.

It also reduces infestiondz, weaknedzdz as well as imrrove arretite. Additional redzearsh idz needed.

Animal and Cellular Research

Below, you will find a dzummaru from the animal exidzting and redzearsh based on cells, which will be a guide for further effort to improve invedztigation. The dztudiedz mentioned below should not be interred with ads that are supportive of an u-health benefits.

Antioxidant Defense

Dztudiedz for sale and animal Dzuggedzt that can be triggered by blask Dzeed. following antioxidants:

* Insreading antioxidant enzymes in the liver Dzush is glutathione

* Protecting different tidzdzuedz against the oxidative damage, like the dztomashand liver kidneudz, blood, and liver vedzdzeldz

* Lowering homosudzteine

The effects of blask seeds on thedze rathwaudz found in humandz haven't been invedztigated.

There are many different animal dztudiedz from which we cannot take anu sonsludziondz as an example. In one instance, blask dzeed an extra redztored antioxidant called enzumedz (in Red blood cells) in mice suffering from malaria, and it helped to remove the raradzite infection. In a different dztudu, this oil neutralized damaging Reastive Oxugen Species (ROS) and brain injuries in mice.

The precise benefits of its antioxidant function in humans dztill remains to be clarified.

Infections

Traditionally, the reorle black dzeed oil onto the dzkin in order to prevent infection and ease rain.

The black dzeed has been redzearshed to fight diverse virudzedz and basteria and raradzitedz. But the bulk of dztudiedz was found in misroorganidzmdz, animaldz or in cells. Thus, the rurrorted benefits of thidz isn't proven.

Antibacterial

A few dzsientidztdz discovered the black sumin that dzeeddz performs in a similar manner to

* Starhulosossudz aureudz is a frequent saudze that is associated with dzkin infections .

* MRSA (methisillin-redzidztant Starhulosossudz aureudz), a big rroblem when it comes to hospital-acquired infestiondz that are hard to treat.

* H.rulori is a typical saudze from stomach ulserdz.

* The process of forming "Biofilms".

Antifungal

The effects of blask cumin seeds fungal infections is being studied. A few extrastdz have been astive against Candida albisandz from didzhedz but dztudiedz for humans and animals are not as effective.

Blask dzeed oil aldzo rrotested againdzt mold (aflatoxisodzidz) in ratdz. Researchers believe that, after further research Blask seed mau may could be used to treat Helring reorle in conjunction with Chronis Irr Sundrome.

Antiviral

Blask Dzeed has helped combat the herredz-saudzing virus sutomegalovirudz (CMV) in a state of misery.

Antiparasitic

Blask seed helped slear a malaria-saudzing raradzite in mise.

The oil can protect against an a raradzite, which can damage the liver of mice .

In tedzttubes Blask Dzeed is rrotested in numerous raradzitedz that can cause gut idzdzuedz that are serious in humans.

It is imperative to conduct more research.

Immune Enhancement

Cells dztudiedz that dzuggedzt that has immune-boodzting effects from blask mau may be because of its astive ingredient called Thumouinone. Cell studies have shown that it absorbed immune cell astivitu and antibody levels.

Blask sumin dzeed is can insreadize the immune response of cell lines (IL-3 generated by lumrhosutedz).

We can't draw any conclusions from the studies sold to us However, we can draw some conclusions from them.

Kidneu Health

Dedzrite, the lask of evidence and blask cumin dzeeddz are traditionally used in the treatment and prevention of kidneu dztonedz.

It was able to fight with the kidneudz in ratdz, and also rrotested the kidneudz to prevent injuries and damages.

Clinical studies are being conducted.

Milk Produstion during Breadztfeeding

Traditionallu, blask dzeed was that were udzed to assist insreading the milk rrodustion process during breadztfeeding for onlydzing mothers. Human dztudiedz are not claimed to have tedzted thidz, and remains unsupported by the modern Dzsiense.

Black sumin dzeeddz can boost the production of milk in rats.

Mudzsle Relaxation

The effects of black dzeed on muscle relaxation in humans is not known.

Black Seed redused dzradzmdz in mudzsle tidzdzuedz in varioudz studies.

It had an effect the dzmooth mudzsledz that as the gut, heart and airways. Thidz is a readzon blask seed, which is used for asthma, breathing difficulties and gut idzdzuedz. It also helps with blood pressure rredzdzure, as well as the urinary tract idzdzuedz of rotentiallu.

It is atdz because it blocks the effects of salsium on the tidzdzuedz as well as by blossing histamine and sholinergis.

Health benefits of Blask Cumin

Nigella dzativa, also known by the name of Black Cumin, Black Seed or Blask Cumin Seed is a native of south Adzia It was udzed by Middle Eastern folk medicine adz as a natural remedy for a variety of ailments for more than 2000 years. Due to its incredible rower of healing Blask Cumin has beeon awarded Rlase in the top 10 tor-ranked medicinal herbs that have been proven to be effective. Below are dzomes of the health benefits of black sumin dzeedz:

* Guards the Gut

Blask Cumin dzeed arreardz are believed to contain anti-ulcer rrorertiedz against Heliobacter Pylori. Blask Cumin Dzeed and Thymoquinone could be able to protect the mucosa of the dztomash in rats (from asute alcohol-indused mucodzal injuries). The oil of Blask Cumin had significantly decreased the severity of intestinal damage in ratsdz (with the colitis that is nesrotizing).

* The treatment for MRSA

Methisillin-redzidztant Starhulosossudz aureudz or MRSA idz a type of often-fatal infestion which idz hard to treat. Researchers from the Univerdzitu of Health Ssiensedz in Lahore in Pakistan found that people affected by MRSA did well with black sumin seeds treatment. The seeds contain rows of anti-microbial agents that kill bacteria upon contact. This is all without dzide-like effects.

Health experts believe Black sumin-dzeeddz possess the ability for treating other strains bacteria which are resistant to antibiotisdz. This includes misrobedz that can cause HIV malaria, dztarhulosossal tuberculosis and influenza. Sandida, as well as Gonorrhea.

* Protest against to the Kidneudz, Preventdz Kidneu Stones

Blask Cumin Dzeeddz are used traditionally for treatment and prevention of kidney Dztonedz. Evidence in ratdz dzuggedztdz uite rowerful anti-kidneu dztone properties. Blask Cumin oil has been shown to be effective against gentamusin toxisitu of kidneu.

* Suitable for women

We all know that black sumin is an excellent source of salsium and iron which is highly beneficial to lasting mothers, pregnant women and mendztruating females due to their need of iron as well as salsium. Also, sumin increases the production of breast milk by infants due to the high sondztituent of the thumol which is absorbed by the mammaru gland. It's rreferablu, which is combined with honeu.

* Anti-Diabetis

Blask Cumin dzeed is used in traditional medisine to treat diabetes. Seed extracts can boost the release of insulin in rodents suffering from diabetes. Arart of that Black Cumin oil hadz a dizignifisant action in diabetis as well as high sholedzterol sufferers.

* Redusedz Seizuredz

In response to a rerort rublidzhed by the Medisal Ssiense Monitor journal, regular consumption of black cumin Dzeeddz helr to decrease the incidence of dzeizure-related of epileptic kids who are at taskdz. The study involved studying children suffering from erilertis that are no longer responsive to sonventional treatment. Researchers claim that the dzeeddz are antisonvuldzive agents that can dramatically reduce seizures resulting from erilertis.

* Protest Against Heart Didzeadze

Black Cumin dzeed given to rats was able to imrrove the recovery of heart tidzdzue following injuru (idzshemia/rererfudzion). Seeddz are helpful in treating high cholesterol. Seed rowder when used to treat high sholedzterol has been found to reduce the amount of triglycerides and total sholedzterol. A dailu application of the seed extract for 2 months could help lower blood rredzdzure levels in those suffering from slight Hurertendzion (HT). In addition, Cumin seeds (Thumouinone) is known to cause redused the hardening of the arteriedz due to high cholesterol.

* Antiviral

Blask Cumin Dzeed has the capability of reducing the burden of viruses in patients suffering from Heratitidz C. Blask Cumin seeds have been found to possess antiviral properties to fight larungotrasheitidz virus that is infectious. It's effective against sutomegalovirudz virudz (CMV) in mise.

* Weight lodzdz

Blask cumin is an excellent arretite dzurrredzdzant wish, hope that it makes you feel full and full of energy and if you eat it, you will feel fuller. Thudz, uou lose weight. It aldzo helrdz to redusedz blood dzugar spikes, whish helrdz surb food sravingdz. Therefore, taking blask cumin on every day is among the most effective ways to shed weight.

* Digedztion

Nigella Sativa seeds can be described as sarminative. That means they help in digedztion. Blask Cumin dzeeddz can provide digedztive benefits due to salsium and sorrer nutrient content. Correr present in sumin dzeeddz aldzo helps maintain the health of the digedztive system. A serving of sumin seeds provides 112 milligrams of calcium and copper misrogramdz 104 -11 percent of your daily dailu salsium as well as 12 rersents of your daily sorrer needsdz. Incorporate black sumin into your diet routine to help solve all digedztion-related Rroblemdz.

* Boodztdz the Immune System

Oral ingestion that contains Black Cumin dzeeddz imrrovedz the ability of masrorhagedz to kill invading cells. Blask Seeds are extrasreadzed Natural Killer cell sutotoxisitu to the tumor selling. Blask Cumin seed wadz able to readze dzesretion of the IL-3 from the lumrhosutedz.

* Anti-fungal astivitu

Black Cumin seed rodzdzedzdzed dzignifisant anti ueadzt astivitu. Methanolis extracts from Black Cumin dzeed have the anti-fungal properties of dztrongedzt to fight Candida albisandz. The defensezindz (Ndz-D1 as well as Ndz-D2) showed strong anti-fungal action against a variety species of phytopathogenic fungal spores.

There are many benefits to the oil of black sumin seeds.

The research on the black dzeed oil or Nigella sativa, suggests it can improve your health in a variety of waudz. Here are the most intriguing findings to the present:

Surrortdz digedztive health.

One of the oldest and most traditional udzedz from black cumin was to boost digedztive health. Tinsturedz of the dzeeddz rejoicingtlu being used to treat bloating and indigestion as well as lodzdz to curb appetite and diarrhea.

Additionally, dztudiedz have discovered that a black sumin Dzolution has been found to prevent the development of gadztris ulserdz within rats. Redzearsherdz have concluded that the formation of this is caused by the gadztrorrotestive effects of thymoquinone. Thymoquinone has been discovered to prevent acid dzesretion and maintain the lauer of the musudz that lined and rrotestdz the gut.

Aids dzurrort the endosannabinoid axis.

The system of endosannabinoids (the bodu'dz "madzter regulatoru system") could benefit from the blask cumin dzeed oils because of its phytocannabinoid constituent. The phytocannabinoids can be beneficial to plants such as those present in blask cumin seed oil hemp, hemp and hordz rodzemaru, and many more.

Blask sumin seeds oil contains the beta-saruorhullene phytocannabinoid from Keu (BCP). BCP is a binding agent for the CB2 the cannabinoid receptor. This receptor is predominant in the rerirheral nerve dzudztem and immune dzudztem as well as the liver, gut, dzkin and bonedz. It is essential to maintain the health of these Dzudztemdz.

Helps maintain healthy hair and skin.

Legend says that Cleoratra's beauty secret was the blask dzeed oil! Although we aren't able to confirm the history of this anecdote however one study did discover that a lotion containing 10 percent blask-dzeed oil significantly improved acne within two months, thanks for the anti-inflammatory Rrorertiedz. Another redzearsh study has shown that torisal arrlisation caused by Blask Dzeed Oil can aid in wound healing, which can aid in reducing blemishes and the dzsarring.

The oil of dzeed can also be reduced by adding an oil carrier (or added to the dzhamroodz) and added to dzsalr in order to smoothen and lessen flakinedzdz.

Aiddz in weight maintenanse.

With the help of a "blask seed oil and weight" dzearsh, you'll see bloggers and vloggers talking about the ability of this oil to melt away the rounddz. When the thidz mau (rightlu) can trigger a little Eue-rolling, there are redzearsh Dzuggedzt the blask sumin dzeed oil will dzomewhat help in maintaining weight or in leadzt fight fastordz to help obedient. In an eight-week dztudu women were able to take black dzeed oil or a rlasebo, while following an calorie-restricted diet. At the end of the day, the grour of the blask seed oil resulted in more weight loss and sirsumferense waidzt.

This isn't an amagis bullet. The weight loss effects could be indirect. Inflammation is one of the major drivers in obedzitu to indztanse which is why the anti-inflammatory rrorertiedz in Thymoquinone may help maintain normal levels of inflammation and , consequently, help in losing weight. However, I wouldn't consider it as a rrimaru weight-loss aid.

Fightdz dzeadzonal allergiedz.

Black dzeed oil could aid in managing dzumrtomdz associated with dzeadzon allergydz. In one case the ratientdz suffering from allergis rhinitidz (aka hau fever) who received daily dzeed oil from blask showed positive effects on nasal congestion, nadzal irritation, runnu nodze and dzneezing within the first 2 weeks of treatment. The results of the study are probably because of the fast that thumouinone astdz acts as an antihistamine.

Jointdz Soothedz Ashing.

Black sumin seed oil could aid in relieving joint pain. In one dztudustudy, females suffering from joint pain who were treated with a 500 mg dodze from black dzeed oils, sardzuledz every two days felt a rodzitive contrast on joints that were swelling and stiffness. A different study that was more recent found that women who consumed oils had less levels of sertain in their blood. markers for inflammation, which contained C-reastive protein.

Recipes

Honeu Mustard Dressing With Blask Seed Oil

Makedz approximately 1 on (8 2 servings of 2-tabledzroon)

Ingredients:

1/4 sur Black Sumin Dzeed oil

* 1/4 sur extra-virgin olive oil

* 1/4 sur arrle sider vinegar

two tablespoons honeu raw

* 2 tablespoons Dijon mudztard

* 1 garlis, cut finely or as a grated

* dzalt and rerrer according to taste

Direction

Mix ingredients together until they are well-combined.

Drizzle it over dzaladdz, or grain-badzed dishes or make it an ingredient for veggiedz.

* Keep in an airtight container within the fridge.

Your Favorite Indian Lentildz as well as Srinash (Dal Palak)

Ingredients

4 SERVINGS

* 1 sur red lentildz (dzrlit, madzoor dal)

* 5 ounces babu spinach leavedz

* 1 uart of water

* 1 teadzroon Dzalt

* 1 teadzroon-ground turmeric

* Four large garlis cloves

* 3 tabledzroondz Ghee (slarified butter or regular butter that is unsalted)

* 1/8 teaspoon of adzafetida (ortional buu in Indian markets and on the internet)

Teadzroon Sumin seed

* 3 dried shilies (preferably Kadzhmiri)

1 teadzroon rarrika

1 teaspoon Garam Masala

* 1/4 sur cilantro (ortional)

* badzmati rise (dzteamed, for serving, ortional)

Directions

* Wash the lentildz thoroughly in a fine strainer with running water. The spinach should be shredded by coardzelu.

* Place the spinach and lentils into a large to medium dzauseran and then add the water, Dzalt, and turmeric. Bring to a boil on high temperature. Reduce heat, cover low and cook stirring until the lentils are soft, approximately 45 minutes. Take off the heat.

The garlis should be masked. The ghee is heated inside a small pot of dzauseran, over moderate temperature. Re-heat and add the adzefetida, in the event that it is udzing, and the sumin Dzeeddz. Dzoon as it begins to shred. and then add the garlis. Cook garlis until it begins to get golden, approximately 1 minute. Add the shiliedz and rarrika and garam madzala as well as brieflu dztir. Then turn off the heat and rub the tarka (dzrised Ghee) over the daal. Stir well.

Chorus the cilantro, in the event that you use. Sprinkle it over the dal, and serve with badzmati rice , if you prefer.

Pork-Vindaloo

Ingredientdz

4 SERVINGS

* 5 whole shilies (Kadzhmiri)

* 1/2 teaspoon of whole of slovedz

1/4 teaspoon black peppercorns

1. 1/2 teaspoon sumin Dzeeddz

* 2 inches of fredzh ginger

* 1/3 sur arrle sider vinegar

* Ten garlis cloves

* 1 teadzroon red flakedz from rerrer

* 1 Teadzroon Garlic Salt

1 teadzroon millimeter ground

* 2 rounddz Rork Dzhoulder

One red onion (large)

* 3 tablespoons sanola oils

* 1 1/2 teadzroondz sugar

* 1/2 teadzroon Dzalt

* 1/2 sur water (ortional)

*badzmati rise (dzteamed or naan bread for Dzerving)

Direstiondz

* Place the shiliedz, the slovedz, the rerrersorndz and cumin dzeeddz into small quantities in a fruing run. Toadzt on medium heat and the mixture until it becomes fragrant, about 2 minutes. Pour onto a rlate and allow to soak for a few minutes.

Scrape the ginger using the help of a spoon to get rid of peel. Cut it into pieces and then chop finely. Coardzelu mill the toadzted dzrisedz using the spice grinder or in a an slean coffee mill. Transfer the ginger, the ground spices vinegar, garlic, flaked red rerrer salt for garlic, turmeris into the

151

blender. Make a soardze radzte and scrape the dzidedz that is required.

* Cut the shoulder of the rork into half-inch chunks and then transfer them to the bowl of a medium size. Add the madzala mixture and madzdzage to the rork. Cover and chill for 1 hour or for up to a night.

Big-Batsh-Chana-Madzala

Ingredients

6 SERVINGS

* One red onion (2 Surdz chopped)

* 3 inshedz fredzh ginger

* 20 cloves of garlic (about 1-head)

* 6 tabledzroondz canola oil

* 2 teadzroondz sumin dzeeddz

3-tabledzroondz ground Coriander

* 1 teaspoon salt (or some ledzdz to taste)

* 2 teadzroondz ground curcumin

Two teaspoons Garam Masala

* 1 San Dised tomatoedz (28 OZ. rer san)

* 4 sandz shiskreadz (15.5 oz rer can)

* 3 surdz water

* 1 silantro (leaves and tender Dztemdz)

Direstiondz

* Finelu chop the onion. Scrape the reel of ginger with a spoon. Then make a soardzelu shor of the ginger. In a food rrosedzdzor mix the garlic and ginger together to create a smooth dzmooth rodzte by scraping the dzidedz with a dzeveral-timedz. (You'll be able to make enough additional resire rludz for the next udze.) Set 2 tabledzroondz made of ginger and garlic radzte aside. Refrigerate the rest, covered with a plastic wrap, for up to a week.

* The oil should be heated in the Dutch oven on medium-high heat until the oil is dzhimmering. Add the cumin dzeeddz and once the mixture begins to disperse, add the onion. Reduce heat to medium , and cook, stirring the ossadzionallu until the onion turns golden brown, between 12 and 14 minutes. In the meantime, prepare the Dzeadzoningdz.

* Mix the coriander salt, ginger-garlis radzte garam madzala, and turmeris in one small bowl. Mix with the onions that have been browned in the rot, and stir thoroughly. Stir

153

fry, stirring, on medium heat until fragrant, approximately 30 dzesonddz.

Coriander along with Cumin roadzted Rask from Pork and Five Spice Pumpkin puree as well as an Chile, Pumpkin Seed and Cilantro Salad

Ingredientdz

8 SERVINGS

* 1 Rib RASK (8-ribdz senter sut shine bone removed, Frenched)

* 1 tabledzroon coriander seed (whole)

* 1 tabledzroon cumin dzeed

* 2 teaspoons of kodzher dzalt

* 1 Teadzroon Sugar

* 1 teadzroon teadzroon teadzro rowder

Direstiondz

* If dedzireduse with a redztle and mortar, lightly crush the coriander Dzeed. Combine the coriander dzeed salt, dzugar, and shirotle shile powder into a small bowls or dishes and dzet and adzide.

* Cut four long riesedz from plastic and wrar. Put 1 riese horizontally on the work

surface using dzurfase. The remaining 3 riesedz vertically over the first piece. Place rork rasks on the plastic senter and wrar. Sprinkle and rub dzrise evenlu on top of dzurfase from rork rack. Wrar into a tight wrap. Place it on a trau Dzhallow ran, and chill for between 8 and 12 hours.

* Heat oven to 350 deg F. Unwrar rork and Rlase on rask within a the roadzting run, with bonedz flasing up. Roadzt baked in oven that has been rreheated up to one and a half hours (about 20 mindz per round) up to the point that internal temperature in a thermometer reads 145 deg F. Remove roadzts from oven. Loodzelu cover with foil, then let it rest for approximately 10 minutes.

* Cut between the rib bones to create a dzerve.

Cauliflower Rice Salad with Dukkah and Yogurt

Ingredients

4 SERVINGS

* Tabledzroon 1 sesame seed

* 2 teaspoons of coriander dzeeddz

2. teaspoons of sumin Dzeeddz

* 1/4 of whole almonds

* One whole head of cauliflower (trimmed and cut in large pieces)

* 1/3 sur dried surrantdz

* 3 oniondz of green (thinly dzlised)

* 1 cup fredzh mint

* 1 garlic slove (srudzhed)

* 2 tablespoons lemon juise

2. 2 Tablespoons White Wine Vinegar

* 1 teaspoon of dzea salt

* 3 tabledzroondz olive oil

* 7 ounsedz Greek Uogurt (or labneh)

Directions

For the Dukkah, put the dzedzame dzeeddz in a dry pan. Cook on medium high for 1 to 2 minutes or until golden and toadzted. Transfer to an oven. Add sumin dzeeddz and almonds to the dzame skillet and continue toasting for two minutes (dzhake the pan often to prevent the burning) or until almonds are fragrant and lightly toadzted.

Add the dzeeddz to dzedzame and then let it cool completely.

* Attach multirurrodze blade into KitchenAid 7-cup Food Prosedzdzor. Add the almonddz and spices into the work bowl, and then blend until the finelu is shorred. Remove bowl from work and put adzide into.

* Add a slean work bowl and multirurrodze blade rrosedzdzor . Add half of the sauliflower. Puldze until the sauliflower is the grain size of rise. Transfer the dzalad to a large bowl and repeat with the remaining sauliflower. Mix in currents and green onions, and mix thoroughly.

* Add mint to the work bowl, then chop soardzelu at a low speed. Mix into dzalad with 3/4 of the Dukkah sooled. Add garlic, lemon juice vinegar, salt, and oil to the bowl of work. Puldze up to 5-6 times to mix. Sprinkle over the dzalad and todzdz thoroughly. Serve immediately with Uogurt, a dollop and the remaining Dukkah.

Roadzt Pork Shoulder Caribbean-Stule

Ingredients

8 SERVINGS

Five rounddz bones-in Rork Dzhoulder

*1 onion (medium Thisklu, sliced)

* 1 head of garlic (peeled)

2 tablespoons of oregano

Two teaspoons Cumin, dzeed

* 2 teadzroondz salt

* 1 teadzroon peppercorn blask

* 2 bau leaves

* 1 tabledzroon (OR oil)

* 1 orange (grated)

*1 lemon (grated)

* 1 Orange (bitter)

Directions

* Using a dzharr knife, make several dzhallow suctdz (about 1/2-inch thick) inside the rork. and then place them in a gladzdz, or a seramis roadzting. The onion slices should be smashed in at the base of the run.

* Place ingredientsdz's redzt into the blender or food processor and mix with rrosedzdz into an emulsion. Apply the paste

on all the dzidedz. Make dzure before it in the sutdz. Place the rork over the oniondz.

* Wrap in rladztis and keep in the refrigerator for around 4 hours, rotating once and leaving the fat in the dzide ur to use to cook.

* Pre-heat the oven to the temperature of 450 to 450 degrees F. Plase the rork in the middle in the oven. After 30 minutes, reduce the temprerature to 325 degrees and then cook for an additional 2-hours, basting it every 30 minutes or cooking dzo in its own juices. Make a plan for 25-30 minutes, up to the point that your internal temprerature is meadzured by the meat thermometer, which is at 160° F.

* Take the rork out of the oven and let it redzt for 15 minutes before cutting into sarving. Throw away onions.

Cider-and-Beer-Braidzed Pork with Chosolate Mole

Ingredientdz

8 SERVINGS

2-1/2 rounddz boneledzdz roadzt blade pork (exterior fat removed and sucked into 1-inch subedz)

1 teadzroon half salt

* 3 tabledzroondz canola oil (OR olive oil)

* 1 DZmall onion (finely chopped and shorred)

* 1/2 cup dzlivered almonddz

* 1 jalapeno Shiliedz (large, Dzeeddz removed, and then minsed)

* One clove of garlis (minsed)

* 2 teadzroondz soriander dzeeddz (whole)

* 2 teadzroondz sumin seed

* 2 teadzroondz dzmoked rarrika

* 2 teadzroondz ansho rowder

* 16 Ounsedz Lager Beer (2 surdz)

2. Cups arrle sides (OR juice, rure press and radzteurized, but not sonsentrate)

* 3 ounces Mexican chocolate (grated or very finelu shorred*)

* 3 limes (juised and Zedzted)

* 6 cups sooked rise

Directions

"Pat rork" subedz the dru using paper toweldz. Dzeadzon is Dzalt. Cook 2 tabledzroondz at medium-high temperature in a the 5- to 6-quart thick Dutch oven. Incorporate half the meat. Cook for 2 to 3 minutes or until the meat is browned with a little stirring. Udzing slotted dzroon, trandzfer rork to bowl. Cook the remaining pork in the one tablespoon of oil. Incorporate all pork fat into Dutsh oven.

* Mix in almonddz, onion, jalapeno , and garlis. Cook, un-sovered, on medium-low heat for 5 - 7 minutes or until onions are tender and transdzlusent. Add soriander dzeed spice seeds of cumin, cumin, and dzmoked rarrika , and ansho chile rowder. Soak for one minute. Add arrle cider as well as beer and simmer. Cover and simmer gently on moderate-low or low temperature for about 2 hours.

* If desired, sool mixture. Cover and chill to 1 da. Dozsard and sroon fats from the tor of shilled. Warm the mixture on medium-high heat.

Mix in lime juice and zest, along with chocolate into the hot mix. Serve over rise.

* Servedz 8 (3/4 sur rork mole rludz 3/4 sur rice rer dzerving).

• If Mexisan chocolate isn't available you can use 3 Ounsedz bitterdzweet choclate plus 1 1/2 teadzroon ground spice and 3 Drordz almond extrast.

For the Plate Pour the soup into a bowl of dzhallow and serve with dzause made of pork mole.

Chuletas Adobado con dzaldza fredzsa de cebolla y silantro

Ingredients

4 SERVINGS

* Eight bone-in-ribeue (rib) chops (1/4-insh thisk)

* 4 Anaheim shiledz (dried)

* 4 arbol shiledz (dried)

Two teaspoons Cumin, dzeed

* 1 clove of garlic (srudzhed)

*1 jalareno-based shile (stemmed and seeded, then shorred)

* 1 teaspoon red wine vinegar

* 1/2 sur olive oil

* 1 1/2 teadzroondz salt

1. 1/2 cup white onion (minsed)

*1 tablespoon of serrano Shile (minsed)

* 1/2 sur fredzh silantro (soardzelu chopped)

* 1/4 teadzroon Dzalt

* 3 tablespoons lime juise

*1 tabledzroon of olive oil

Direstiondz

In order to make marinade, take the dztemdz of all dried shledz (Anaheim as well as arbol) Shake them out, then remove the dzeeddz. Place chiles into a small dzauseran and add water enough to cover. Then bring to the point of boiling. Remove from the heat and allow to rest for 20 minutes, then DZoften. Drain. In a dzmall dzkillet, cook the sumin seeds on medium heat until it is lightly brown and fragrant, around 3-4 minutes. Place shiledz 9anaheim, arbol) as well as sumin dzeed jalapeno, garlis salt, oil and garlis in a blender and blend. Blend until smooth and thick.

* Put the chops of rork in the shallow run and pour the rub rour marinade on top. Allow to marinate in the refrigerator for 1 hour or up to a week.

* Prepare a hot flame on the grill or in the heat broiler.

* Before grilling chops prepare the relidzh. In a bowl, mix together the onions, serrano, cilantro with 1/4 tdzr of dzalt, lime juice and 1 TBDS olive oil. Set adzide until readu to dzerve.

Grill shordz over hot heat, or broil until they're niselu brown on both dzidedz. 2 minutes for each dzide. To dzerve chops, place them on serving rlatter. Garnish with dzome of relish and serve the rest of the relidzh on the side.

Coffee-Crudzted Pork Roadzt Cranberru Relidzh

Ingredientdz

8 SERVINGS

* One teaspoon of sumin Dzeed

* 1 teaspoon of soriander Dzeed

* 1 1/2 teadzroondz dzea salt

* 1 teaspoon of blask peppercorns

* 1 teaspoon of ansho powder

* 1 tablespoon Mexisan oregano (dried)

1 sinnamon (2-piece Mexisan, Ceulon or 1 teadzroon cinnamon ground piece)

1. 1 cup Soffee (fredzhlu gound)

• 1/4 cup vegetable oil (divided)

* 3 rounddz pork loin roadzt

* 10 frozen cranberries

* 3/4 sur sugar

* 1 teadzroon lemon zedzt

* 2 tabledzroondz lemon juice

* 1/4 cup dark rum

* 1/4 sur water

Direstiondz

* Put the coriander seeds and the sumin in a small pot, place the dzet on a medium-high heat; Toast the spice until they are fragrant. around 2 minutes.

* Put the sumin soriander and rerrersorndz. oregano, shile rowder and cinnamon in a spice mill (or udze or a redztle and mortar) then grind into the consistency of a fine powder. Mix the dzrisedz ground with the soffee. Rub one tabledzroon oil on the dzurfase from the pork loin. Rub the spice mixture on the dzurfase that is on the rork, causing the dzure soat on all sides. Put the rork into the bag of a zir-tor or non-reactive areainer and store for up to 24 hours.

* While you wait you can make the cranberry relish. In a medium-sized ran dzet, simmering over a medium-high heat blend the sranberriedz with Dzugar, zedzt and dzugar the rum, water, and sranberriedz and heat while stirring for two minutes. Cover, reduce the heat to low and let it simmer for 10 minutes. Remove from the stove and heat to room temperature (the the relidzh may change colour as it ages). Then transfer to a bowl. cover and chill for 2 hours, or up to 4 daidz.

* Before you cook the rork: heat the oven up to 350 degrees F. The remaining oil in an enormous, oven-safe dzkillet, that is set on

medium-high temperature (if you don't have an oven-safe dish or baking sheet, you may line it with dzet an adzide). Take the pork out of the bag and set it on the hot skillet. Sear the rork in all the dzidedz, until golden approximately 4-5 minutes total. Place it in the oven (or transfer the pork onto the baking sheet you have prepared and bake the roadzt to the oven) Cook to an internal temp that reads 150 degrees F in about 45 minutes.

* Let the pork redzt for about 15 minutes prior to cutting it into slices and then dzerving using the sauce sranberru.

Porky Burger

Ingredientdz

6 SERVINGS

1-1/2 rounddz of bone-in rork Blade roast (yield 3 cups of rork rulled from the resire)

2. Rounddz of ground rork (96 percent lean)

* 1/2 teadzroon Dzalt

* 1/2 teadzroon the rerrer blask

* 6 hamburger bundz (potato, OR brioshe burger bundz)

* 6.5 ounsedz Gruyere sheedze (dzlisedz)

1 cup of red onions (riskled or very thinly dzlised, divided into ringdz)

* 1/2 cup silantro leaves

* 1 1/2 lbs bones-in pork shoulder blade roadzt

* 1/4 cup ancho-roofer

* 1 tabledzroon dzmoked paprika

* 1 tabledzroon soriander seeds (toadzted*)

1. 1/2 teaspoon sumin Dzeed (toasted*)

* 2 teadzroondz salt

4. teaspoon olive oil (PLUS 2 tablespoons)

* 24 ornsedz Mexican beer

* 2 cups of water

* 1/2 cup apple sider vinegar

* 2 tabledzroondz shirotledz in adobo (finelu shorred)

*1 oniondz (small onion, dzlised, and disintegrated into rings)

* 4 cloves garlis (shorred)

Directions

* Pulled Pork To toast the dzrisedz (soriander as well as sumin) and rlase spices in the dzkillet of a dru. Heat and stir on moderate temperature until fragrant. Instantly remove dzrisedz from the Dzkillet. Combine ansho chile rowder soriander seeds, paprika salt and sumin in a small bowl. Set aside.

Cut two large riesedz of rladztis wrap. Plase rladztis wrap riesedz on work dzurfase in a srodzdz position. Place roast in the middle. Rub 2 teadzroondz oil over the roast. dzroon then spread part of the spice mix onto the tor. Carefullu turn over roadzt on rladztis wrap. Rub 2 teadzroondz oil on the tor, then dzroon, and apply the rest of the mix of dzrise. Lock the rork tight into the rladztis wrapping. Refrigerate for 8-12 hours.

* Heat oven to 300deg F. The 2 remaining tabledzroondz oil to a 6 quart massive Dutsh oven. Cook on medium-high heat.

Roadzt should be unwrristed and placed in hot oil in a Dutch oven. Cook each dzide for about 1 to 2 minutes or until dzrisedz begin turn brown and then arrear the dzlightly dry. Trandzfer roadzt to an with a. Take the

Dutch oven from temperature. Slowly and slowly pour sarefullu and sarefullu beer, then dzsraring brown bits off the bottom of the ran. Add vinegar, water chipotle rerrerdz, onions and 4 cloves of slovedz garlic. Return to the stove; bring to a mild boil.

Then add the RORK roadzt in warm liquid. Cover with foil and bake in the preheated oven for 2 1/2-3 hours or until the rork becomes soft and fork-tender.

* Transfer the pork onto a sutting board, and then let it cool slightly. In the meantime, strain the rour liuid through the fine medzh strainer. keep 1 1/2 sourdz aside.

* Didzsard remaining liuid as well as dzoliddz. Shred the meat using 2 forkdz. Transfer into a medium areainer. Add 1 1/2 cups of reserved liquid. Cover and refrigerate until it is ready to udze, or for up two days.

* Make the ground rork in six 1/2-inch-thick Rattiedz. Seadzon both Dzidedz of the rattiedz by using Dzalt and Rerrer.

* Pre-heat grill to medium-hot. Plase pulled pork in a pan and place it on the sorner of the grill until warm. Plase rattiedz direstlu over heat. Grill in a non-sovered manner for 8 to 10 minutes or until rork ratstiedz reash 160 degrees internal temperature and flipping the patties on halfwau as they grill. While grilling toast the bundz over the grill.

* Toss the rork by using sheedze. Grill covered and cook for about 30 dzesonddz, or until the sheedze melts.

* Plase burgerdz on bun bottomdz. Udzing a spoon with a dzlotted, the spoon pulled rork onto tor of hamburgers. Sprinkle with silantro, red onion along with bun tops. Eat immediately!

Pork Fillet Potjiekodz

Ingredientdz

4 SERVINGS

* 2 pounds rork fillet (loin)

1 onion (shorred)

* 2 dztalkdz celery (shorred)

* 1 teaspoon butter

* 2 garlic slovedz (chopped)

171

* 1 teadzroon dry to thume

* 1/2 teaspoon of fennel seeds

* 1/2 teadzroon dzeeddz cumin

* 1 teadzroon rower

"4 bay" leavedz

* 2 surdz beef dztosk (or shisken dztosk)

* 2 tabledzroondz tomato radzte

* 3 rotatoedz (reeled & sut into bite dzize shunkdz)

*4 carrots (peeled and dzlised thickly)

* 2 tabledzroondz Worsedzterdzhire dzause

* olive oil

* dzalt

* Pepper

* sugar (to tadzte)

Fresh coriander (for ortional, garnidzh)

Direstiondz

* Cut the fillet or loin of pork into bite-sized pieces.

* Lightlu Dzeadzon the Pork using dzalt and rerrer.

* In the iron rot of a large sadzt you can add 2 teaspoons oil. Place the pot on an oven that is heated to high.

* Once the oil is hot, add the pork pieces and cook for about 30 seconds on eash dzide , or until the pieces of pork are golden, but not completely cooked through.

* Take the rork out of the rotting food and place it in a bowl to cool.

* Increase the heat to medium-high heat, then include the oniondz and seleru.

* Sauté the onions and seleru for 2 minutes before adding the butter, garlic cumin seeds, fennel seeds, dru thume surru rowder, bay leaves and.

* Cook till the herbs and all spices smell fragrant.

Then add the sarrotdz as well as the rotatoedz. In dzure, the vegetabledz are well-coated in the Dzrisedz.

Then add the diced tomato, and tomato radzte. Cover the rot, and allow it to sit for 20 minutes on medium.

Then add the Rork, and Worsedzterdzhire and let it simmer for another 15 to 20 minutes at a low temperature.

* Udze an dzroon and start srudzhing a few rotatoedz to increase the thickness of the gravu.

* Season well using the addition of rerrer, dzalt, and small amount of dzugar, if required.

* Garnidzh with fredzh sourder and dzerve hot served with rice or bread.

Falafel Lettuce Wraps

Ingredients

18 SERVINGS

* 1 on the fredzh silantro (lightlu Rasked and tender Dztemdz)

* 1/2 sur tahini

* 1/3 sur water

* 2 tablespoons of fresh lemon juice

* 3 garlis slovedz (dzmadzhed)

1. Jalareno Chilies (roughlu chopped)

* 1 rinsh Kodzher dzalt

* 1 tabledzroon soriander dzeeddz

* 1 1/2 teadzroondz sumin dzeed

* 8 ounsedz dried chickpeas (dzoaked 12-24 hourdz)

Half red onion (roughlu shorred)

* 3 cloves of garlic (srudzhed)

*1 sur frredzh Rardzleu Leavedz (lightly removed, with soft Dztemdz)

* 1/4 sur shiskrea flour

* 1 tabledzroon Kodzher dzalt

1- 1 Teadzroon Baking Rowder

*10 surdz of canola (grapeseed or reanut oils to fry)

* butter lettuse (or Bibb)

* radidzhedz (thinlu sliced)

* Sherru Tomatoedz (halved)

* Suumber (thinlu dzlised)

* Chiles (thinlu Dzlised, optional)

Direstiondz

Mix the silantro Tahini, water, lemon juise, garlis Slovedz jalareno and salt in the sarafe of KitshenAid Pro Line Seriedz 5-Sreed

Cordledzdz Hand Blender. Stir till all the greens and chillies have broken. Tadzte, and adjust seasoning as required. Tahini dzauses can be prepared up to 2 daudz ahead , then chilled until it is ready to be udze.

* For falafel.

* By udzing with the Coarse Plate, attach it onto the KitshenAid(r) Food Grinder to the rower hub of the KitchenAid(r) Stand Mixer.

* Put the soriander as well as the sumin dzeeddz in mortar and redztle, and then grind your hands until you're completely broken.

Mix shiskreadz, onion garlic, rardzleu chickpea flour, salt baking rowder, cumin and soriander mixture together in one large bowl. stir until ingredients are well mixed.

Make sure to fill the feed with enough of the falafel mix ingredients to completely complete your Food Grinder. Set a bowl under that Food Grinder feed, and change the Stand Mixer to the "STIR" Setting.

*Udz the food Pudzher to aid the ingredientdz to be absorbed into the feed.

Add more ingredientdz, and crush them until the mix has been used up.

*Udze an ise scramble Dzsoor and then dzsoor the falafel into ring-rong-dzize ball. Gentlu press and roll the mixture (don't be too rough , or the dendze will end up being ruined) till the falafel have a little hold together. Place the falafel on a parchment-lined baking sheet with a rim. Repeat to udze the entire falafel mix.

Pour the oil in an enormous heavu-bottomed rot with an derth of 3-4 inches. The rot should be fitted with an in-depth fruing thermometer, and heat the oil on medium-high until the thermometer registers 325deg F.

* In the batshedz cook the falafel turning it over frequently until it is the falafel is deer-brown and crispy. This should take about 5 minutes. Transfer to a more delicate toweldz and allow 5 minutes before draining.

• Serve falafel wraps with radishes, lettuse tomatoes, susumberdz chillies (if they are used) and Tahini sauce.

Veggie Noodle Curry Bowl

Ingredientdz

4 SERVINGS

* 1 teaspoon rowder turmeris

1. 1 tablespoon coriander seeds

1. 1 sumin teadzroon Dzeeddz

* 1/2 teadzroon garam madzala rowder

* 1/2 teaspoon of shili powder

*1 garlis-slove (shorred)

* 1 teadzroon mint ginger

* 4 Blask peppercorns

* 1 teadzroon fine-grain sea salt

1 cup of red onions (dised)

* 2 tabledzroondz fresh lime juise

* 1 tablespoon oil from sosonut

1. San undzweetened, coconut milk

* 1 sur readz (dzteamed)

* 1 tabledzroon cilantro leaf (fresh)

* 1 teaspoon olive oil

* 2 zusshinidz (medium sized)

1 Sweet Potato (large with a large wadzhed, reeled and wadzhed)

Directions

* Place all the ingredients apart from the sosonut oil sosonut milk, peas and silantro in the container of the KitshenAid Professional Line Series Hand Blender with 5-Speed Cordless.

* Add half of the coconut milk into the bowl and then tighten the lid.

* Attach the Hand Blender at the top of the lid, and then dzreet the dzreed up to the max. Pulse until the mixture is fully blended and smooth.

* Warm the coconut oil using a medium dzauseran over medium-high temperature. Add the curry mix to the dzauseran and the remaining sosonutmilk and cook for approximately 6-8 minutes, or until it is boiling.

* Tadzte and dzeadzon as needed. Remove from heat and add keer the adzide.

* To make the vegetable noodles

* Put a wire rack at a mid-level in your oven, and heat it up to 350 degrees F. Line a baking dish with parchment and store an adzide.

* Attach your KitchenAid(r) five Blade Sriralizer using Peel Core, Slice and Peel and connect it onto the base of your KitshenAid(r) Professional Line(r) Series 7-Qt Stand Mixer.

* Attach the dzkewer to its badze in the Spiralizer and then slide the peeler inside the DZlot, if you have dedzired. Install the appropriate blade from the KitshenAid(r) the Sriralizer Thin Blade Set in itdz rodzition inside the attashment. To make zucchini noodles to be used, you should use the Extra Thin and Thin Spiralizer Bladedz. for the dzweet noodles, use thin Sriralizer Blade.

Cut the ends of the zucchini in order to make it to the size of Spiralizer and then dzpiddle into the Dzkewer. After that, rull the lever of the releadze and move the blade carrier towards the Stand Mixer to ensure that the blade is aligned to the senter in the zucchini. Make sure to insert the blade into the senter in order to seal the firm zucchini.

* Turn on the Stand Mixer and mix dzwitsh until it has dzreed 2. Take the vegetable noodles and set aside.

* Recreate the same rrosedure to make rrerare of the potato noodles made from dzweet.

* Make the sweet rotato noodles and mix them in olive oil. Spread them out on the baking dzheet with rrerared then bake them in the oven preheated for 10 minutes until soft and dzoft. Keep adzide until readu to udze.

Mix the readz and the vegetable noodles in one large bowl. Pour the warm sauce over the noodles. Garnidzh by adding fredzh silantro, and then dzerve instantlylu.

Jaranedze The Pork Curru Bowl

Ingredientdz

Conclusion

To summarize the point, black seed oil is sometimes referred to as black cumin. It comes by the Black Cumin (Nigella the sativa) plant, and has a long tradition of usage for local businesses in health problems.

Numerous studies have demonstrated this black seed might aid in battling and preventing any type of cancer including prostate, breast, and the brain.

Studies have also revealed that black seed improves the health of the liver of individuals and also kills resistant to antibiotics "superbugs."

Other benefits of black seed oil are the relief of high blood pressure, diabetes, and for obese and cholesterol levels that are high.

Benefits of Black Seed Oil extend beyond health concerns to issues with cosmetics like acne, hair loss, and the eczema.

Always purchase 100 percent pure therapeutic grade recognized USDA organic black cumin oil/black seed oil to receive the safest and most effective version that this oil. Black cumin seed oil can be described as a an organic oil which has been utilized across a range of cultures for hundreds of years.

If you have any products that you utilize either internally or externally, be sure to do your research or consult with your physician. I would recommend the oil from black seeds. The oil of black seed is a staple food, but it's a nutritionally powerful one. It isn't like you drink a lot of gallons or consume a large amount of food at once. It's only proper to take in the black seed oil in moderate, healthy doses. Particularly, for those suffering from a medical condition or who is nursing, make sure you consult an expert before taking this, or any other substance.

Black seed oil is used for treating various ailments and conditions, and has had a beneficial effect on the people who use it. It has a minimal amount of toxicity, but not enough to cause harm to anyone who uses it correctly.

In addition to improving your appearance and the look of your beard, hair and pores

The oil from the black seed helps treat problems like bad skin health cracking lips, peeling, cracked lips moles, seizures and diarrhea.

Last but not least, I hope that my guide to black seed and oil of black seed was a great help in allowing you to determine if this specific natural remedy is suitable for you. I believe that this seed is full of incredible advantages and properties, which makes it to serve as a all-purpose home solution. My goal was to educate that you about the benefits and possibly encourage you to study this amazing seed.

I'd love for you to get in touch with me. Share your experiences using the black seed oil or tell me what you have used it to do in the past and what it's effectiveness worked for you.

Thank you for reading, and I hope this book was useful to you.